Table of C

Prescription for Type 2 Diabetes: Exercise

by Milt Bedingfield MA, CDE

Edited by Debbie Voiles

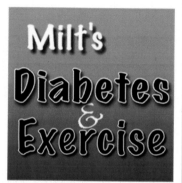

Milt Bedingfield, MA, CDE
Clinical Diabetes Educator
Exercise Physiologist

TheExerciseDiabetesLink.com
MBedingfield@yahoo.com

813-569-9243

or online book retailers.

Printed in Victoria, BC, Canada.

ISBN: 978-1-4251-6335-8 (sc)
ISBN: 978-1-4251-6336-5 (eb)

*Our mission is to efficiently provide the world's finest, most comprehensive book publishing
service, enabling every author to experience success. To find out how to publish your book, your
way, and have it available worldwide, visit us online at www.trafford.com*

Trafford rev. 3/31/10

Trafford PUBLISHING® www.trafford.com

North America & international
toll-free: 1 888 232 4444 (USA & Canada)
phone: 250 383 6864 ♦ fax: 812 355 4082

Introduction:

When I had nearly finished writing this book, the publisher suggested I would find a book with a format I liked that we could use as a pattern for my book's format. I went to the bookstore and looked at books already written about diabetes. I pulled an armload of books off the shelf and began going through them. Then I continued my search at home on the internet. At one well-known web site I found 27 books about type 2 diabetes. Fifteen of them had titles that related to food or diet such as: diabetic exchanges, carb counting cookbooks and one-pot meals. The titles of the remaining twelve implied that they were overall guides to diabetes.

I could not find a single book with exercise or physical activity in the title, not on the internet nor in the bookstore. Although surprised, I shouldn't have been, because for as long as I have been a diabetes educator and even before that, the focus of treating diabetes has focused on nutrition, modifying what the person with diabetes is eating. Although very important, there is far more to successfully managing diabetes than food selection and reduced serving sizes.

In the hospital based education program where I work, people frequently want to come in for a Basics of Nutrition class or sign up for a nutrition consultation with a dietitian, mistakenly believing that learning how to eat better is all they need to do to take care of their diabetes. Unfortunately, that's not enough.

As we continue to look for better ways to treat type 2 diabetes, more and more research studies are showing that the performance of regular exercise plays a significant role in not only the treatment of type 2 diabetes but also in its prevention.

This book will discuss some of this research and explain why being more physically active and getting regular exercise is at least as important, if not more important, than dietary modifications.

Acknowledgements

I wish to thank Mr. Phil Rossiter for his expertise and generosity and for donating his time to create many of the illustrations in this book.

I also want to thank Debbie Voiles for editing this book and for all that she taught me along the way. Carole Cambridge and Mila Appolinario, both nurses, were very influential, and mentored me when I was just getting started in the field of diabetes.

They taught me just how important it was for people with diabetes to receive the best education possible. For this, I will always be greatful.

Thank you to my parents, Milt and Julie Bedingfield, who were both instrumental in me writing this book. They have always been very supportive and encouraging in all of the projects I have been involved.

I would like to give a special thanks to my family, Terra, Chelsie, Natalie, Maggie, Adryana, and Daniel who provide constant inspiration for everything I do.

Illustrations

Susi Galloway Newell and
Phil Rossiter

Cover Design by Debbie Voiles

Dedication

I want to dedicate this book to the memory of my younger brother, Chris and my older sister, Laurie. Both of their lives ended before they were able to accomplish the goals they had set for themselves and live their dreams.

About the Author

Milt Bedingfield, a native of Tampa, Florida, earned a BA in Biology from the University of South Florida in 1980 and an MA in Exercise Physiology in 1988. He began his career as a diabetes educator in 1993 at University Community Hospital in Tampa, and in 1995 became a certified diabetes educator.

Over the 16 plus years Milt has been a diabetes educator, he has taught hospitalized patients, individually, as well as outpatients in the classroom setting. From 2000 to 2006, Milt supervised an outpatient exercise facility designed specifically and exclusively for people with diabetes. During that time, Milt was fortunate to observe, firsthand, the incredible results patients achieved after exercising for just a few short months.

After seeing the amazing transformations in patients' overall health, particularly as it pertained to their diabetes, Milt was motivated to get the word out as to just how effective exercise is at improving the lives of patients with diabetes. Milt has felt for many years that exercise is understated as a means of diabetes management, when in fact, it just may be the single most effective means of controlling the disease. This was the motivation that led Milt to write this book.

Chapter 1
How People Develop Diabetes

Before one of our comprehensive classes was to start one day, a class that was expected to last until about 3:00 pm, a middle aged gentleman got the attention of one our educators and motioned for her to come over to where he was sitting. As she approached he gestured for her to lean over closer to him as if to indicate that he didn't want anyone else to hear what he was about to say.

"I need to find out how long we are really going to be here today. I know when I registered I was told that the class would go until about three o'clock. We are not really going to be here that long are we?"

The instructor grinned and replied, "Yes sir, class typically runs until about 3:00, sometimes 3:30." This was an answer the man was not at all expecting and he appeared quite surprised. Thinking their conversation was over, the instructor turned away and went back to what she had been doing.

A moment later she was being summoned again, "Psst, psst, excuse me, Ma'am?"

She again stopped what she was doing and walked over to where the man was sitting. The man motioned with his hand for her to come even closer. She did, and in a much quieter but very obviously frustrated voice the man told her, "Listen, the reason I asked you that is because I own my own business, a rather large lucrative business; I have over 150 employees working for me, and I really cannot afford to sit in this class all day. You know what I'm saying?"

His tone suggested that he expected her to sympathize and agree with him. Not so. That is not the kind of thing you say to a diabetes educator, not one who has seen the life altering effects of poor diabetes control.

This time the instructor, very deliberate in her actions, turned and squared off directly in front of him. Locking her elbows and placing her hands flat on the table, she leaned over close to the man, looked him straight in the eyes, and said, "Listen, you need to understand something here, this is diabetes we are talking about. It is unfortunate that you have to miss work to be here today, but whether you have a small company of twenty or a $50 million company, you need to be here so you can learn how to take care of your diabetes. Do you know what I'm saying? She was very stern and not smiling.

Surprised that the educator didn't see it his way, the man seemed to be searching for what he could say next to bolster his argument. Sensing this, before he had a chance to continue, she said, "Let me put it another way; if you want to stay healthy so you can keep running your business, you need to learn how to take care of your diabetes."

That comment proved to be the knockout punch. The patient took a deep breath and sighed, "Yes, ma'am."

Although not what the patient wanted to hear at the time, he has since credited this instructor with turning things around for him. If I remember correctly, I believe this patient refers to this instructor as "the lady that saved my life."

It has been my observation that a large majority of patients who show up for class have no idea of the severity of their illness. Those that do recognize the seriousness of diabetes usually do so as a result of seeing the devastating effects poorly controlled diabetes has had on their friends or relatives.

One of the first things I do when I walk into a new class of patients is ask how many of them would rather be somewhere else today. Usually at least half of the hands go up. With some there is no hesitation, as if to say, "Heck, no, I don't want to be here." Others raise their hands with some hesitation, a little sheepishly. These people are a little embarrassed to admit they would rather be somewhere else.

After acknowledging their responses, I raise my hand; they look surprised. "What, you think diabetes is my only interest?" I respond.

"I'm only here because my wife made me come!" shouts out one man.

"My doctor's office signed me up for the class and said I better show up or he was going to make me start taking insulin shots," remarks another lady.

Fortunately, to balance these comments there are those who respond, "No, I wanted to be here; I just got diabetes last month and I don't know anything about it."

A lot of patients who end up in a diabetes class are there, not because *they* want to be there, but because *someone else* wanted them to be there. I have found that person is usually the doctor or a spouse. As a result, these patients are not necessarily ready to learn yet and may not get as much out of the class as they could. Fortunately, many of these people change their attitude sometime during the two days of class and leave with a much greater understanding of the disease, along with a willingness to accept and treat it.

Imagine trying to put one of your child's Christmas presents together without instructions. Last Christmas Eve I remember sitting on the floor struggling to assemble a dinosaur community. I was constantly referring to the instructions, and even then it took an hour and a half to connect all of the pieces together in the right sequence.

In that scenario, if I connected two of the wrong pieces, I could disconnect them and start over with no harm done. But what about with diabetes? What if you make mistakes taking care of it because you don't really know how? Are these mistakes harmless? Some mistakes may not be serious, but others may be *very* serious.

Inappropriately treating low blood sugars and not knowing how to take care of your diabetes when sick are just two examples of situations that can be very dangerous.

Just as I needed instructions to put the dinosaur community together, patients with type 2 diabetes need instruction regarding how to care for the disease. You simply can't take care of your diabetes if you don't know how.

If someone tries to manage their diabetes with minimal or no instruction, controlling the disease is likely to be so difficult and frustrating that they may just give up and stop trying. The result could be catastrophic.

Everyone with diabetes needs instruction because there is simply so much that needs to be learned. I usually recommend patients attend a formal group class. Those for whom group classes may not be appropriate are patients who may have significant problems hearing, seeing, concentrating, or sitting for extended periods of time. For these patients one on one teaching usually works best.

For everyone else I believe group classes work best for several reasons. One big reason I like a class setting is that you have the opportunity to ask questions. You also benefit from other people's questions and comments, and the class participants can actually serve as a source of support for one another. It is interesting to see a group of people who were total strangers at the beginning of day one carrying on and exchanging phone numbers at the end of class the second day. These people, who vary widely as to level of education, economic situation and age, find common ground in their diabetes. When they leave to go home after finishing the second day of class some may come to realize that there are a lot of other people faced with the inconvenience of having diabetes and that there are people worse off than themselves. Perhaps the best reason for attending a diabetes class or series of classes is the way patients are shown how everything they have learned about diabetes fits together like a puzzle and that each part of the treatment, or each piece of the puzzle, has its place and is important.

For those of you who don't have the opportunity to attend a diabetes class, at least you are fortunate to have this book, the next best thing to a class, and in some cases, maybe even better. I have tried to write this book the same way I teach class, using the same examples, following the same order and emphasizing the points I believe to be the most important.

Why I Wrote This Book

I suppose you have heard the expression, " Necessity is the mother of invention."

It couldn't be more true. When I think about what motivated me to write this book I think about that phrase. In this case, it was a lack of focus on three of the topics that I believe to be crucial in the management of type 2 diabetes.

In my 15 years of teaching patients about diabetes, I have never been able to find in patient literature, nor have I heard any diabetes educator or physician explain to patients with the necessary emphasis or enthusiasm, the need for exercising diligently and making exercise the cornerstone of diabetes treatment.

I have become increasingly frustrated by the lack of attention exercise and physical activity receives as they pertain to treating type 2 diabetes, particularly in light of the research that unequivocally supports it. I believe that in too many cases, instead of health care professionals engaging their patients in a serious discussion about the need for regular exercise and how it can significantly improve their blood glucose control, the suggestion of exercise seems to be mentioned so casually and with such little enthusiasm that the patient may feel as though they can take it or leave it, that doing exercise or not doing exercise was not going to have much impact on their diabetes either way.

Well, this is not the case and definitely the wrong message we would like patients with type 2 diabetes to go away with. This book will inform patients with type 2 diabetes about just how significant a role exercise plays in the treatment of their diabetes. In fact, I want patients to know that the absolute best thing they can do for themselves, and their diabetes, is exercise diligently and lose excess body fat.

Please understand here that I said body fat, not body weight, as there is a big, big difference.

Additionally, more emphasis should be placed on patients keeping a closer eye on their blood pressure, total cholesterol, low-density cholesterol, high-density cholesterol and triglycerides. All of these, when elevated above normal levels, constitute major cardiovascular risk factors that in large part are responsible for two out of three people with diabetes dying from either a heart attack or stroke. (1) (www.diabetes.org/heart disease-stroke.jsp)

In some instances, when someone is informed of their diabetes, lowering their blood glucose levels becomes the main and sometimes only focus, resulting in less attention being afforded to the so vitally important cardiovascular risk factors.

With the unusually high prevalence of heart disease and stroke in patients with type 2 diabetes, it is crucial that patients maintain good control of their cardiovascular risk factors. Patients should strive to avoid even temporary lapses in control of their cardiovascular risk factors. It is unfortunately true that for patients with type 2 diabetes, maintaining good blood glucose control is not enough to adequately care for the disease. It also requires controlling *all* of the cardiovascular risk factors.

The third reason for writing the book is that I have also come to realize that there were many people with long standing diabetes who really didn't understand the illness, what probably caused it, and how to best treat it.

These people *think* they understand what is wrong with them but they really don't. They think they know what led to their diabetes, but many times they don't. They think they know where their focus should be, that is, what they should focus on to take better care of their diabetes, but they really don't. In this book I will explain to patients exactly what is wrong with them and the probable cause of their diabetes in a way they can easily understand and remember. I keep it simple and lighthearted. Although diabetes is a very serious illness, learning about diabetes doesn't have to be overly technical, scary and unpleasant.

Sometimes patients come up to me after class and tell me that after seeing my presentation they now have a much better understanding of what's going on with their pancreas, specifically their beta cells, and what insulin resistance is all about. They also tell me that they plan to get out and start exercising again, that they were unaware as to how helpful exercise could be in managing their diabetes.

I'm hopeful that everyone who reads this book will come away with a far better understanding of both type 1 and type 2 diabetes and the integral roles both exercise and fat loss play in successfully managing the illnesses.

It is important for anyone diagnosed with any illness or disease to make every effort to understand the disease as best they can. I feel strongly about this because successfully managing diabetes frequently requires patients to make sacrifices, to do some things they may not be accustomed to doing and in many cases don't want to do. An example might be enjoying a bowl of ice cream before bed. If it is suggested to the patient that they only eat the ice cream a couple times per week instead of every night and they understand the rationale behind reducing the ice cream, it may be easier for the patient to make the change.

Must Know Info

Type 2 diabetes is very serious. Anyone who tells you otherwise is poorly informed. Successfully managing type 2 diabetes requires nearly constant attention and effort to avoid complications. Successfully managing diabetes also requires knowledge of the disease. Knowing what to do and what to avoid in order to keep blood glucose levels in check, and knowing how to take care of your feet and what to do if you have an unusually high or low blood glucose reading are just several of the things essential to know.

In fact, there is so much for the newly diagnosed patient to learn, it is recommended that all patients newly diagnosed with type 2 diabetes receive 10 hours of education within the first year of diagnosis. This is the amount of training generally considered necessary to be adequately prepared to take manage diabetes.

This book will explain in detail the sequence of events that most likely led to the development of your type 2 diabetes as well as the two *most important* things you can do to successfully treat it. Although I will discuss other aspects of diabetes care, such as blood glucose monitoring, medications, nutrition, hypoglycemia (low blood sugar) and foot care, you will quickly see that the main thrust of the book is on how weight loss (actually fat loss), and the appropriate type and amount of exercise can so positively impact type 2 diabetes.

Diabetes and Termites

One Saturday morning several years ago, on my way to the kitchen I noticed something peculiar about the molding above my front doors. There was a six-inch section of molding just above the point where both doors meet where if I didn't know better I'd think someone had punched it in with their fist.

In disbelief I walked up close and felt the molding with two fingers. What was left of the wooden molding in that spot crumbled and fell to the floor. You see, just underneath the paper-thin layer of wood was nothing but air. Termites had quietly and methodically eaten away the wood beneath the surface.

Curious to see if the termites had done any more damage, I felt to the left and to the right of the spot. Although the surrounding molding looked to be unaffected by the termites, I was surprised to see that when I poked on that area, it too collapsed, having nothing but air behind it.

After carefully probing all of the molding around my front doors, it turned out that all of it had been at least partially chewed on by the termites. In fact, I found that some of the termites were just sitting down for their next meal when I discovered them. What was most surprising was how, except for that one six-inch section of molding, the rest of the molding around my front doors had appeared to be fine, until I pressed on it when it then collapsed. Without poking at the molding you would never have known that the termites were destroying the wood around my door because on the surface everything looked fine. It was only after the termites had really done a lot of damage beneath the surface layer of wood that I noticed there was a problem.

This same scenario can be applied to diabetes. People will often take their diabetes casually, particularly if they don't notice feeling any different after they develop diabetes than they did before. When they hear that having abnormally high blood sugar levels will cause damage to many of their organs, they rationalize that somehow their bodies must be different because even with high blood sugars they still feel fine. They somehow believe that their bodies can handle the higher levels of sugar in the blood, like they have a higher threshold for sugar or something. After all, how could all those terrible complications happen when none of the affected body parts or organs ever hurt?

Consider this situation. Let's use you as my example. One day you wake up and your foot feels funny, like it is asleep or something. However, after breakfast, with teeth brushing and all grooming chores complete, your foot is still tingling, feeling somewhat numb. You misdiagnose yourself as having a pinched nerve from sleeping wrong and move on with your day.

Two days later your foot still feels peculiar and so you go to your doctor. After thoroughly examining you, the doctor says the problem sounds like neuropathy, damage to the peripheral nerves of the body caused by high levels of sugar in the blood. A review of the blood tests done at the doctor's office that day also indicates that there is some protein in the urine. This indicates that your kidneys are starting to become affected by the higher than normal amounts of sugar in the blood.

Later the same week, when you are at your eye doctor for an annual exam, the doctor sees some damaged capillaries in the back of your retina. This, the doctor informs you, is known as retinopathy.

Amazed at all the things the doctor has found wrong with you, you ask, "How come all of these things are going wrong with me all of a sudden?"

The doctor replies, "These complications did not develop overnight; they have been progressing from a stage when you don't usually notice them to the point, now, when you cannot ignore them. These complications have been coming on since the day the blood sugar levels first rose above normal. All of this time when you felt fine, under the surface, deep inside your body, these complications were getting started and gradually getting worse until, eventually, they became severe enough to notice."

You see the similarity between the termites and diabetes? Termites and higher than normal levels of sugar in the blood are both destructive. Termites gradually eat away at the wood until the damage is so great that the building eventually crumbles. But early on, when the termites are first getting started, their destructive work goes unnoticed. With diabetes the increased levels of sugar in the blood can initially damage small capillaries in various organs, going unnoticed. At this point the patient feels fine, mistakenly thinking this diabetes is no big deal. Eventually, however, somewhere in the future when the damage to the capillaries becomes severe enough, the patient begins to feel the pain and discomfort of the complications. Similarly, when the termites do enough damage, it becomes obvious the wood has been under siege by the termites.

The worst and most frustrating part of all of this is that once complications are present, the damage that has occurred to the organs will never go away. Regardless of how well you take care of yourself from then on, even if you become the model patient, the complications that are present will be there forever.

I stress to my patients in class in the strongest terms I know the importance of taking care of their diabetes right from the start. Even when the complications are already present, I emphasize the need for good diabetes control, as it is likely to prevent the complications from getting worse.

Now for the Good News

For most people with diabetes, their disease is completely controllable. What this means is that although diabetes is very serious, if you learn what you need to do to take care of it and you do that, there is a good chance you may be able to avoid developing any of the life altering complications and can live a long and healthy life.

The life altering complications I am referring to are neuropathy, damage to the nervous system, retinopathy, damage to the retina of the eye, and nephropathy, damage to the nephrons of the kidney.

These are commonly referred to as microvascular complications or complications that result due to damage being done to the smallest blood vessels in the body, the capillaries. Neuropathy can develop early in the course of diabetes, and is sometimes already present when the diabetes is diagnosed.

Neuropathy, usually first seen in the feet, is described as a burning, tingling, or throbbing, in the feet or toes, either intermittently or all of the time. Eventually, neuropathy can lead to partial or total numbness in the toes, feet, and legs, and in some cases it may contribute to the need for amputation of an extremity. Additionally, neuropathy is the primary cause for the impotence frequently encountered among type 2 patients who are unable to maintain good blood glucose control. Typically, eye disease, or retinopathy and kidney disease, nephropathy, do not occur early on and may take as long as ten to fifteen years to develop.

In retinopathy, small capillaries in the back of the eye, the retina, become damaged due to the elevated levels of sugar in the blood. This damage can cause them to rupture or leak. Treatment for retinopathy is aimed at stopping the bleeding and restoring good blood glucose control. With nephropathy, the nephrons of the kidneys become damaged and cannot filter the blood effectively. Eventually, as the nephropathy progresses, the ability of the kidneys to filter waste from the blood is so limited that help is needed. This is when dialysis becomes necessary. Once dialysis is initiated in a patient with diabetes, it is very likely the patient is already living with most, if not all, of the other diabetes related complications, including heart disease. Although these complications are not likely to kill you, at least not right away anyway, they can certainly have a tremendous impact on the quality and length of your life.

It may be hard to imagine that any good could ever come from being diagnosed with diabetes. To the contrary, I have seen in many cases, cases where patients were highly motivated to effectively manage their diabetes, where their overall health actually improved after the diagnosis. How could this be? As a result of making the lifestyle changes usually necessary to successfully manage diabetes, excess body fat is often shed frequently leading to a lowering of blood pressure. In addition, blood levels of the harmful, artery clogging, LDL cholesterol are likely to drop while levels of the artery protecting HDL cholesterol are likely to go up. The reduced body fat and blood pressure as well as the improvements in blood cholesterol levels all reduce the risk of heart disease.

Developing Diabetes

What I would like to do now is explain how you probably developed your diabetes.

I have found that a great many people who have diabetes, even those who have had it for quite some time, do not understand the disease and what all is involved. It is important for you to understand the way most people develop diabetes and what the root causes are. Knowing this, I believe will make it easier for you to make some of the changes in your life that you may need to make to control your diabetes.

In the next several pages I will explain what happens in a normal situation, that is, how normal blood sugar levels are maintained. I will then explain what goes wrong when you develop type 2 diabetes. Later in the book I will explain what goes wrong when you develop type 1 diabetes; however, since the focus of this book is type 2 diabetes, I will postpone the discussion of type 1 for now.

Let me start off by introducing the players. (Please refer to the accompanying series of pictures).

Introducing the Players

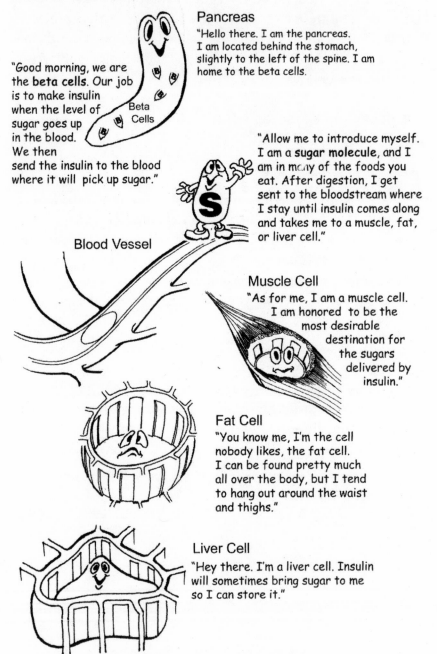

Pancreas

"Hello there. I am the pancreas. I am located behind the stomach, slightly to the left of the spine. I am home to the beta cells.

"Good morning, we are the **beta cells**. Our job is to make insulin when the level of sugar goes up in the blood. We then send the insulin to the blood where it will pick up sugar."

Beta Cells

"Allow me to introduce myself. I am a **sugar molecule**, and I am in many of the foods you eat. After digestion, I get sent to the bloodstream where I stay until insulin comes along and takes me to a muscle, fat, or liver cell."

Blood Vessel

Muscle Cell

"As for me, I am a muscle cell. I am honored to be the most desirable destination for the sugars delivered by insulin."

Fat Cell

"You know me, I'm the cell nobody likes, the fat cell. I can be found pretty much all over the body, but I tend to hang out around the waist and thighs."

Liver Cell

"Hey there. I'm a liver cell. Insulin will sometimes bring sugar to me so I can store it."

Meet the players involved in controlling blood glucose levels

The boomerang-looking organ on the left is the pancreas. In an area of the pancreas commonly referred to as the "Isles of Langerhans," you will find the beta cells. It is the beta cells that are responsible for insulin production. Insulin is a life-sustaining hormone made of protein, and it is this hormone that facilitates the entry of glucose into various tissue cells throughout the body. (Insulin will be discussed in far more detail in the medications section of the book.) I think of the beta cells as little insulin producing factories.

To the right of the pancreas, and continuing down somewhat below the pancreas, you will see a blood vessel. This vessel represents just one of the many vessels inside the body. The S's you see in the top portion of the blood vessel represent sugar molecules in the blood. Moving to the right of the blood vessel you will see a muscle cell, a fat cell and a liver cell.

We are going to say that the two S's in the vessel represent a fasting blood sugar level of 90mg/dl. A fasting "blood sugar" is when the blood sugar level is tested when no food or drink has been consumed in the past eight hours. A normal fasting blood sugar is anything less than 100mg/dl. Mg/dl are units of measure used when quantifying the amount of sugar in the blood. Mg. is the abbreviation used for milligrams, while dl. is the abbreviation for deciliter. So a blood glucose reading of 90mg/dl means there are 90 milligrams of glucose in one deciliter of blood. A deciliter is one tenth of a liter and a liter is approximately one quart.

Keep in mind now that in the first illustration and explanation I will be explaining what goes on in a *normal* situation, the way things are supposed to work in someone who does not have insulin resistance and diabetes. I will use myself in this example.

Proper Working Order or How Things Are Supposed to Work

In this example, let's begin by saying I have a fasting blood sugar level of 90mg/dl. Imagine that for breakfast I have an average size bowl of cereal with a cut up banana and milk. This breakfast looks to be made up of mostly carbohydrates or sugar. Taken individually, the cereal is mostly broken down to sugar, the banana is all sugar, and there is sugar in the milk.

The sugar from all three of these sources enters the bloodstream. As the level of sugar in the blood starts to rise, a message is sent from the blood vessels to the beta cells telling them to get busy and start making insulin.

The beta cells respond according to how much sugar enters the blood. If a lot of sugar enters the blood as a result of eating a meal high in carbohydrates or starch, then a lot of insulin will be made, and if only a little sugar enters the blood, the beta cells will make much less insulin. It is important to keep in mind that, in reality, carbohydrates and starches are sugar. Carbohydrates and starches will be discussed again later, but for now, just keep in mind that they both turn into sugar when digested.

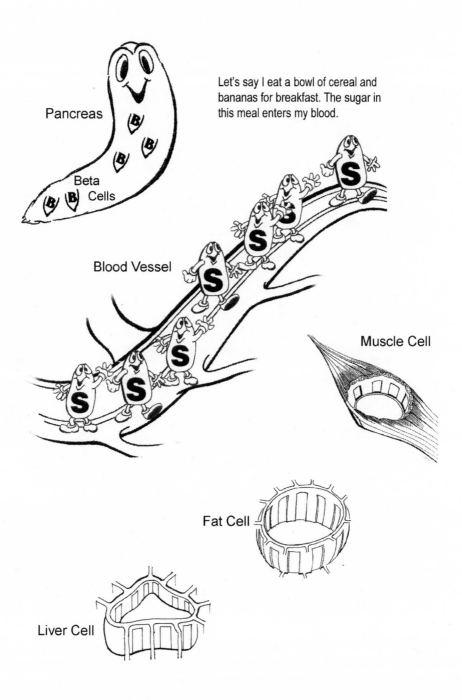

Pancreas

Beta Cells

Let's say I eat a bowl of cereal and bananas for breakfast. The sugar in this meal enters my blood.

Blood Vessel

Muscle Cell

Fat Cell

Liver Cell

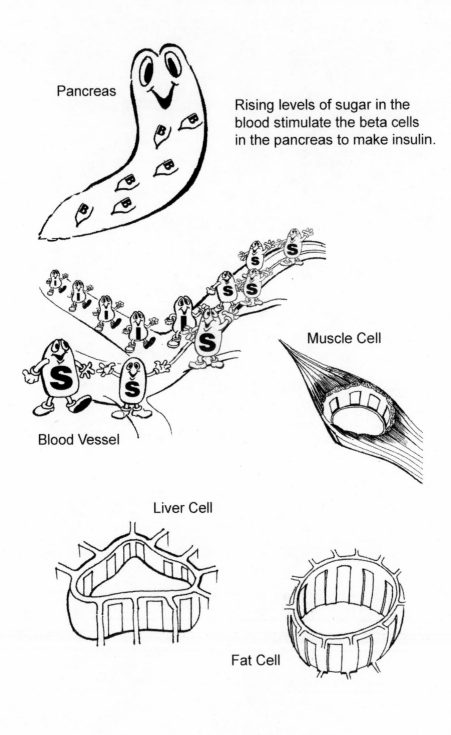

Pancreas

Rising levels of sugar in the
blood stimulate the beta cells
in the pancreas to make insulin.

Muscle Cell

Blood Vessel

Liver Cell

Fat Cell

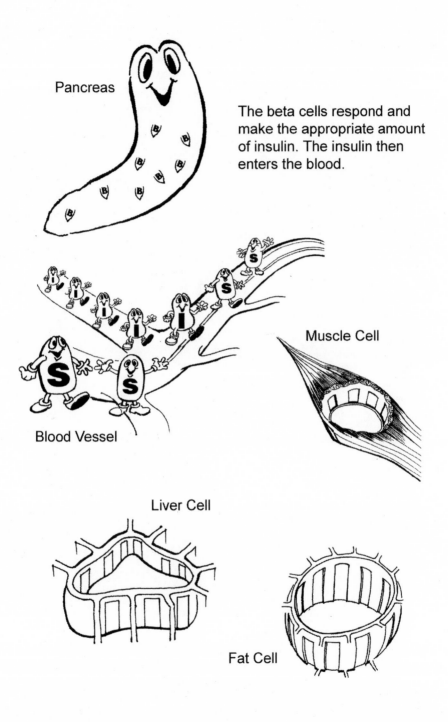

Pancreas

The beta cells respond and make the appropriate amount of insulin. The insulin then enters the blood.

Muscle Cell

Blood Vessel

Liver Cell

Fat Cell

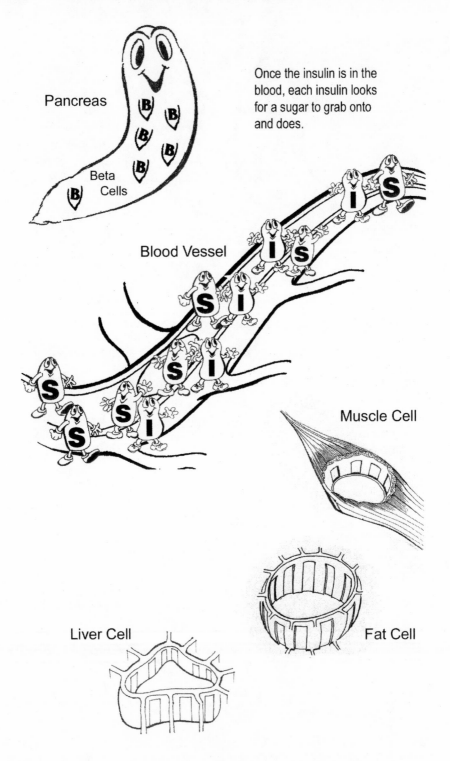

Once the insulin is in the blood, each insulin looks for a sugar to grab onto and does.

Pancreas

Beta Cells

Blood Vessel

Muscle Cell

Liver Cell

Fat Cell

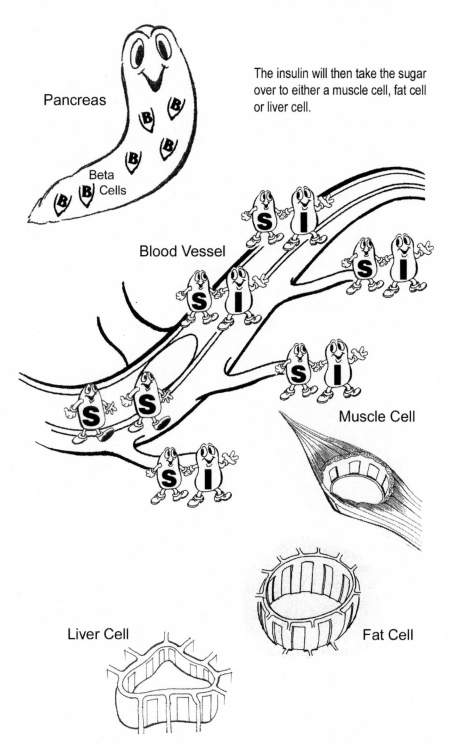

Pancreas

Beta Cells

The insulin will then take the sugar over to either a muscle cell, fat cell or liver cell.

Blood Vessel

Muscle Cell

Liver Cell

Fat Cell

Each cell has many, many doors that open and close to let nutrients into the cell and waste products out of the cell. The insulin opens a door to the cell and escorts the sugar inside.

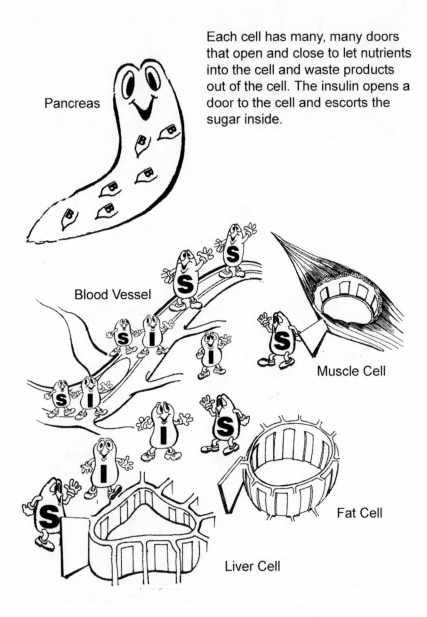

Pancreas

Blood Vessel

Muscle Cell

Fat Cell

Liver Cell

Once the insuln takes the sugar out of the blood and helps it into the muscle, fat, and liver cells, the level of sugar in the blood returns to pre-meal levels, resulting in a sharp decrease in the amount of insulin produced by the beta cells. This illustrates the way things are *supposed* to work.

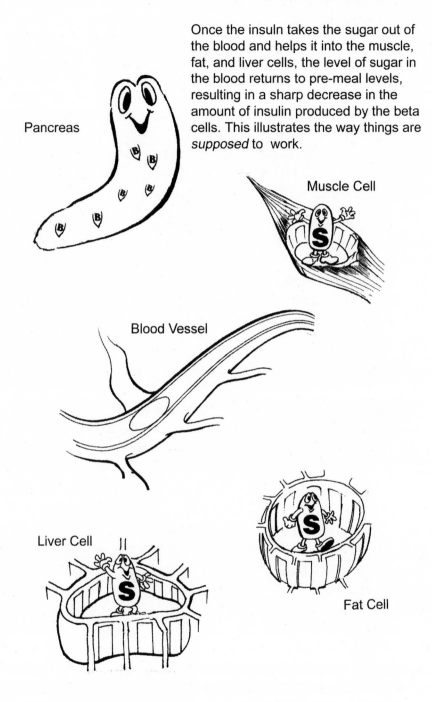

Pancreas

Muscle Cell

Blood Vessel

Liver Cell

Fat Cell

Once the insulin is made, it is sent to the blood stream with instructions to find a sugar molecule and grab hold of it. After the insulin has found a sugar and grabbed hold of it, it then takes the sugar to a muscle, fat or liver cell.

Let's say that in this case, the insulin takes the sugar to a muscle cell. The insulin, while still holding onto a sugar, finds one of the many doors on the cell, knocks, and asks the voice on the other side if it is okay to open the door and escort the sugar inside the cell. The same thing happens with the fat and liver cells.

I like to think of the insulin as a UPS delivery person. They pick up a package at one location and then deliver it to another location. Then they're done! That's essentially all insulin is doing, picking up sugar that's in the blood and then taking it where it needs to go, to a muscle, fat or liver cell. Technically, insulin goes one step further in that insulin also acts as a doorman opening the door to the cell so the insulin can enter.

If things are working properly, most of the sugar that enters the bloodstream is removed from the bloodstream rather quickly by the insulin and deposited in various muscle, fat and liver cells. The amount of sugar remaining in the blood is the amount that is needed for normal brain function and for activities of daily living. It is important to mention here that only insulin is capable of picking up sugar from the blood and taking it to the muscle, fat and liver cells, then facilitating its entry into the cell. Without insulin the sugar would remain trapped in the blood. The only way any sugar could ever get out of the blood would be when it was filtered out by the kidneys and ended up in the urine. This would be likely to happen when the level of sugar in the blood reached approximately 180- 200mg/dl. At levels this high the kidneys realize there is a problem and will try to help reduce the amount of sugar in the blood by filtering some of the sugar from the bloodstream. Unfortunately, though, the kidneys are incapable of removing enough sugar from the blood to maintain normal levels.

Now, getting back to the story, let's say that, as an example, the beta cells need one hour after every meal to make the insulin necessary to clear all of the excess sugar out of the blood. Suppose I eat only three times a day or three meals a day. If this were the case, my beta cells would only work for three hours a day, one hour after each of my three meals. On those occasions when I eat more than three meals a day or when I do a lot of between meal snacking, my beta cells would obviously have to work much longer to make the necessary insulin.

Conversely, if there were times when I went for long periods without eating, my beta cells might almost shut down, as the need for insulin would be very minimal. An important point to make here is that in a normal situation the beta cells work for a while, making the necessary insulin needed after meals, and then are able to rest for a while between meals when far less insulin is needed.

That's it. That's the way it is supposed to work. The blood sugar level never really has a chance to climb very much in the normal situation because the sugar is being removed from the blood by the insulin and deposited in the muscle, fat and liver cells at about the same rate at which it is entering the blood from the intestines.

It's the same thing as if you try to fill a bucket full of water when the bucket has a big hole in the bottom. As soon as the water enters the bucket, it runs out of the hole in the bottom, thus never allowing the level of water in the bucket to rise.

Enough about me, now let's talk about you.

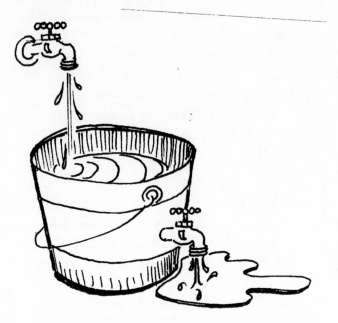

As long as the amount of water entering the bucket is approximately the same as the amount of water leaving the bucket the level of water in the bucket will change very little. Similarly, the level of sugar in the blood should never really climb very much, even after eating, if the amount of sugar entering the blood is similar to the amount of sugar being removed from the blood by the insulin.

Now I will explain the chain of events that leads to the development of type 2 diabetes in the vast majority of cases. If you have diabetes, which I may assume you do if you are reading this book, there is a good chance that this is how you developed it.

When Things Go Wrong

Think back to the day you were diagnosed with diabetes. For the purposes of explanation let's say you were diagnosed June 1st 2006. Now go back five years before that. That puts us at June 1st 2001. This is when it all started, where the story begins.

I think it was a Tuesday. Let's say when you woke up that morning your blood sugar level was a healthy 75mg/dl., a completely normal reading. Remember, Mg/dl represents milligrams per deciliter. Now you eat your breakfast. You had a bagel with cream cheese and a large glass of milk. Bagels are virtually all carbohydrate, or sugar, all of which will enter your blood stream after digestion. There is little to no sugar in the cream cheese; it is mostly fat with some protein. The milk contains sugar, protein and fat, all of which will enter the bloodstream.

So far, so good, everything is normal. As soon as the sugar from the meal starts getting into the bloodstream a message from the blood is sent to the beta cells in the pancreas telling them to get busy and start making insulin. The beta cells respond and start making the necessary insulin. The insulin is transported from the beta cells to a major blood vessel where the insulin enters the bloodstream. Upon entry into the blood, the insulin molecules grab hold of some sugar.

Once the sugar is firmly in the insulin's grasp, the insulin molecule carries the sugar to a muscle, fat or liver cell. Upon arrival at the cell, in this case a muscle cell in the right thigh, the insulin looks for a convenient door to open so it can escort the sugar inside.

After a suitable door is found the insulin knocks on the door and asks permission to bring the sugar inside.

"Yes, by all means, please, open the door and come in. I have been expecting you," says the small voice coming from inside the cell.

The insulin reaches for the handle on the door and turns it, simultaneously pulling back on the handle. This is when something very peculiar happens. The door doesn't open! The insulin repositions its grip on the door handle and tries again. Still nothing. The door doesn't budge.

Understandably puzzled and frustrated, the insulin turns around and leans back against the cell door thinking of what to do next. After all, nothing like this has ever happened before. Up until now the doors have always been quite easy for the insulin to open. Looking for some answers, or what to do now, the insulin pulls his cell phone out of its holster and calls the pancreas.

"Hello, this is the pancreas speaking, how may I direct your call?"

"Can I speak to one of the beta cells?" asks the insulin.

"Just a minute and I will connect you," says the pancreas."

There must have been a lot of calls coming in to the pancreas that day because the insulin had to wait several minutes to be connected. During the wait time the insulin was informed the conversation might be taped to ensure customer satisfaction. The insulin was okay with that.

"Hello, this is Bart, one of the beta cells, speaking, how can I help you?"

"Bart, I am an insulin you guys made about a half hour ago and I got a problem."

"How can I help you Bart?"

"I'm over here in Betty's right thigh muscle, about two inches above the knee, and I can't get the door to the cell open."

"Hmm, have you tried any of the other doors?"

"Well, no Bart, if I had gotten in through another door, I wouldn't have needed to call you now would I?"

"Okay, calm down, we'll get this worked out. Go to another door and try to open it."

"Okay, hold on, I got to set the phone down. Listen, if we get disconnected it's because my battery is running low. Okay, hold on, I'll go try another door.

Nope, no luck it doesn't want to open either."

"Hmm."

"Do you know what the problem is and can it be fixed? I gotta get this sugar into the cell."

"I know. I'm going to try to help you out. First of all, I can tell you that you are not alone. I have already received about a dozen calls this morning from other concerned insulin all over the body that can't get the doors to the cells open, some from as far away as the feet. If you give me your exact location, we are in the process of making some additional insulin and we will send one your way and see if that helps get the door to that cell open. Just hang in there, and we'll try to get that insulin over to you just as soon as we can. We are getting word that many of the doors to many of the muscle, fat and liver cells are becoming resistant to opening.

Okay, I'm showing that another insulin is on its way to your location and should be there in two and a half minutes. His name is Marvin. When he gets there, explain to him that you need help getting the door open and he should be able to help you with that, okay? Can I do anything else for you today?"

"No, I just needed help getting that door open."

"Okay, well you have a nice day and thanks for calling Beta Central."

As promised the beta cells make additional insulin, enough to send another insulin molecule to all of the cells where the doors have become difficult to open.

With the help of the additional insulin, the doors that were difficult to open can now be opened allowing the sugar to enter the cell. As a result the extra sugar that entered the blood from the last meal can now be taken from the blood by the insulin and carried to muscle, fat and liver cells throughout the body, reducing the level of sugar in the blood to near pre meal levels.

The blood sugar level never gets a chance to really rise too much above pre meal levels because, shortly after the sugar starts to enter the blood from the meal, it is removed from the blood by the insulin and deposited in the muscle, fat and liver cells.

The difference between what is happening now and June1st, 2001, the date I said was 5 years prior to the onset of diabetes, is that a majority of the body's muscle, fat and liver cells now require twice as much insulin to open the doors to the cells. If, hypothetically, the beta cells work for an hour after each meal to make the necessary insulin, and three meals a day are eaten, then the beta cells would work for three hours a day.

In this case, however, if the beta cells have to produce twice as much insulin per meal, then the beta cells would be working for two hours after each meal or about six hours a day instead of the usual three! From this point forward the beta cells reprogram themselves to produce twice as much insulin as in the past every time they are stimulated to make insulin.

It has always been the policy of the beta cells to do whatever is necessary, within their means, to facilitate the entry of sugar from the bloodstream into the appropriate tissues of the body, even if it means making increased amounts of insulin.

In the future, cell doors become even more difficult to open and increasing quantities of insulin are needed. Beta cells find themselves working three, four, and eventually five or six times longer than they had ever worked before! Some beta cells may be observed working nearly round the clock in order to make sufficient insulin to get the doors to the cells open.

Until one day one of the beta cells collapses just minutes after sending his last insulin to the bloodstream. The stress of having to make more and more insulin, year after year, day in and day out, has finally caught up with this little guy. The beta cell never regains consciousness and to this day remains in a comatose state.

Initially thought to be an isolated event, this was to be only the first of a long line of casualties resulting from the beta cells' hard work. With more and more beta cells becoming dysfunctional, sometimes two or three per night, this meant even more work for the remaining, nearly exhausted, beta cells still able to function. After all, these beta cells were not only doing their job but also trying to pick up the slack created by the untimely demise of their colleagues.

As usual, bad news travels fast, and when word of the rapid decline in beta cell function spread, calls from concerned beta cells from across the country began pouring in to the pancreas, offering words of encouragement and support. It was a result of conversations with other beta cells that led to a surprising discovery.

It is not normal for a beta cell to give out, becoming dysfunctional, even when asked to make increasing amounts of insulin. It seems that even when beta cells are overworked due to insulin resistance, there are many beta cells out there that never become exhausted to the point of becoming dysfunctional.

Insulin resistance is the technical term used when the normal amount of insulin cannot get the doors to the cells open and greater amounts of insulin are needed, making greater demands on the beta cells, just what I have been discussing over the last several pages. So why is it that some beta cells can handle the increased workload without becoming exhausted and dysfunctional and others cannot?

The answer lies in the genes. DNA testing performed on a large number of the consenting dysfunctional beta cells reveals that there is a genetic aberration or mutation that prevents them from working as well as they should. These beta cells have a genetic defect causing them to become dysfunctional when stressed or overworked as in the case of insulin resistance. This genetic problem may have been passed to them from their parents or they may have even developed it themselves. Regardless, these cells are in a sense handicapped or crippled and lack the ability to work long hours without breaking down and ceasing to function.

As an example, perhaps you were just diagnosed with type 2 diabetes. It may be that you inherited genes that instructed your beta cells to shut down once they were asked to work more than 18 hours a day. The guy next door who is 54 percent body fat and eats, sleeps, eats and watches television all day, has beta cells that work pretty much all day; However, these beta cells never received genetic information from a blood relative instructing them to shut down when asked to work more than a specified amount. In the absence of some genetic abnormality, beta cells should be able to work for long periods without ever becoming dysfunctional as is my example of the person that is overweight and sedentary, (insulin resistant), but does not develop diabetes.

Once about 50 percent of the beta cells have stopped functioning, there are not enough beta cells left to make sufficient insulin to get a lot of the doors to the muscle, fat and liver cells open. As a result, much of the sugar that should have left the blood stream and entered the muscle, fat and liver cells remains trapped inside the blood vessels.

With nowhere to go, the levels of sugar in the blood begin to rise above normal. This is the true onset of diabetes.

It is important to remember that until approximately 50 percent of the beta cells have stopped functioning blood sugar levels will remain normal. It is generally believed that beta cell function continues to decline the longer someone has diabetes. As an example, for patients that have had diabetes for a long period of time, it is likely that far less than 50 percent of the beta cells are still functioning, as they should.

Unfortunately, unless something is done to make life easier for the still functioning, but very fatigued, beta cells, they are likely to exhaust themselves, eventually, and become dysfunctional as well. It is conceivable that someday, if the patient has diabetes long enough, all of the beta cells may have had time to wear out and become dysfunctional. This is most likely to occur in a person that is diagnosed with diabetes earlier in their life versus later in their life.

Insulin Resistance

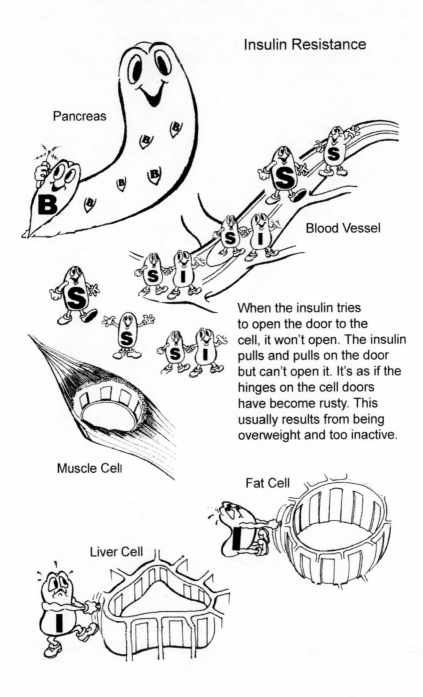

Pancreas

Blood Vessel

Muscle Cell

Fat Cell

Liver Cell

When the insulin tries to open the door to the cell, it won't open. The insulin pulls and pulls on the door but can't open it. It's as if the hinges on the cell doors have become rusty. This usually results from being overweight and too inactive.

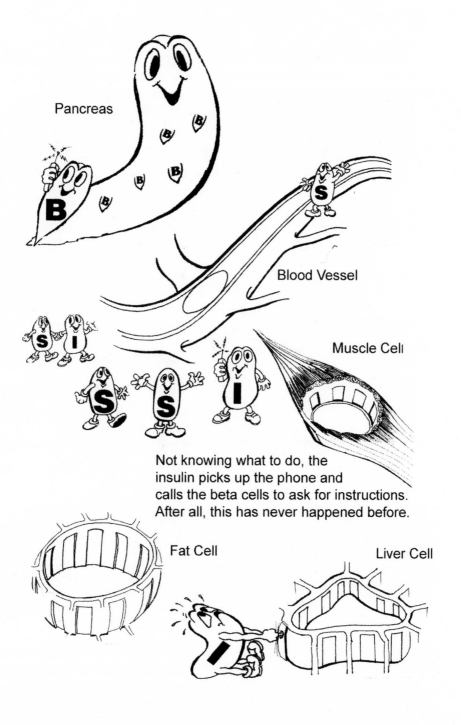

Not knowing what to do, the
insulin picks up the phone and
calls the beta cells to ask for instructions.
After all, this has never happened before.

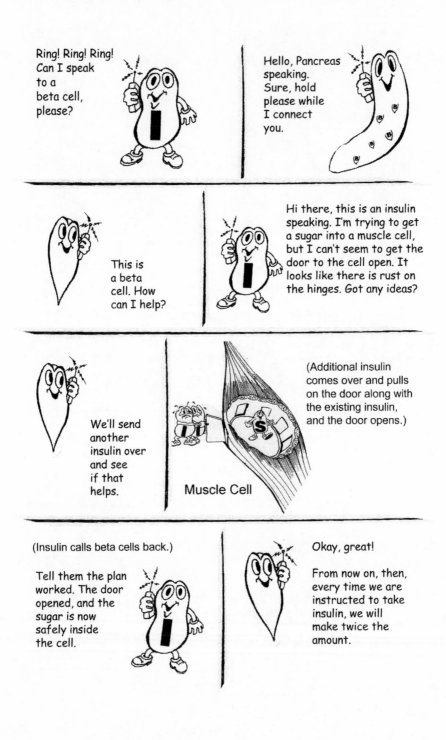

Working together, the insulin gets the doors open and the sugar enters the cell. The blood sugar level returns to normal. As long as the beta cells are willing to make enough insulin to get the cell doors open, the blood sugar level will continue to be normal.

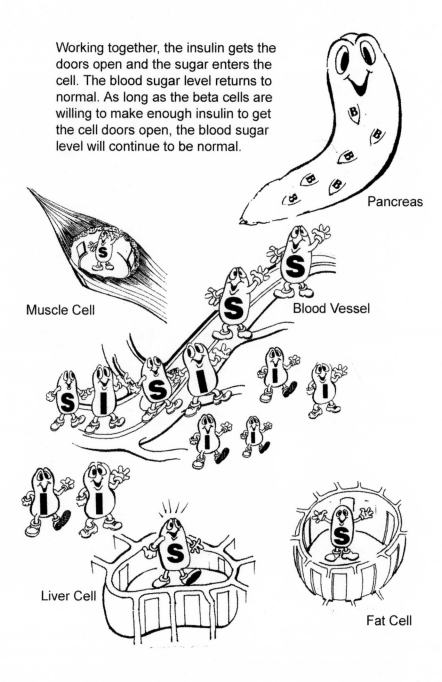

Pancreas

Muscle Cell

Blood Vessel

Liver Cell

Fat Cell

Pancreas

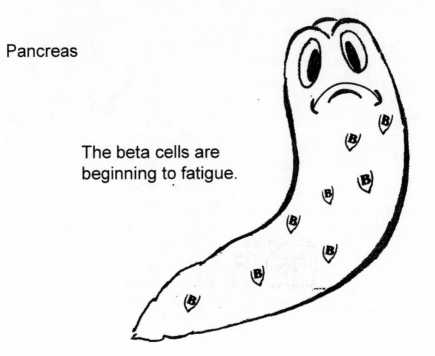

The beta cells are
beginning to fatigue.

If patients continue to be overweight and inactive,
the rusty hinges on the cell continue to get worse
and worse, causing the beta cells to make more
and more insulin every year.

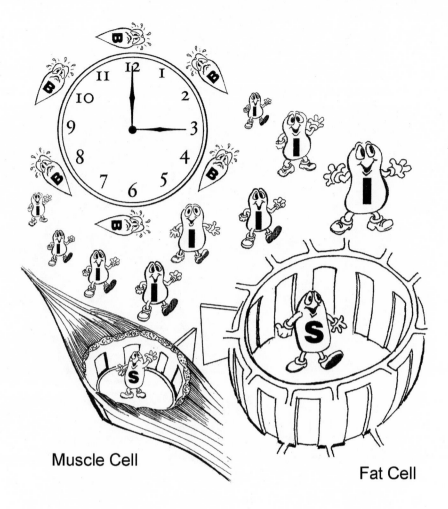

Muscle Cell

Fat Cell

Eventually, the beta cells, many near exhaustion, are working nearly around the clock in order to make enough insulin to get the cell doors open so sugar can enter.

Pancreas

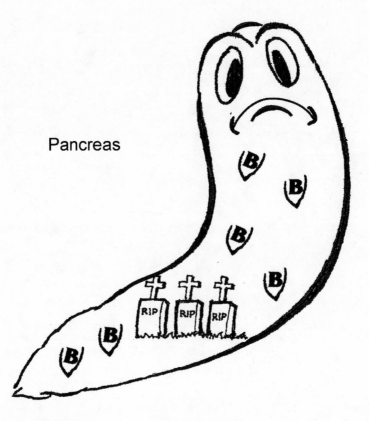

Until one day, when about 50 percent of the beta cells quit, never to work again; they actually become dysfunctional and die.

Once this happens, there are no longer
enough beta cells to make sufficient
insulin to get many of the insulin resistant
doors open. Sugar accumulates
in the blood, leading to abnormally high
levels indicative of diabetes.

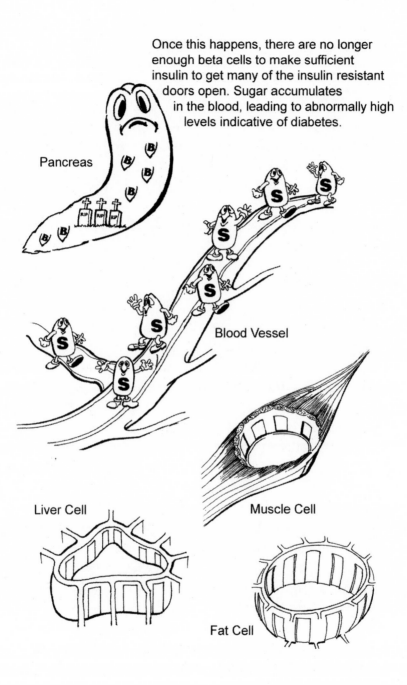

Pancreas

Blood Vessel

Muscle Cell

Liver Cell

Fat Cell

What I have just described here is the typical sequence of events leading up to the development of type 2 diabetes. As I mentioned previously in this section, it is known as insulin resistance and is the cause of type 2 diabetes about 80 percent of the time.

You may have heard your doctor mention the term insulin resistance when explaining to you how you developed diabetes. Many times it takes more than one explanation before it is understood. As an example, patients sometimes become confused because they are thinking, "Wait a minute, I thought my doctor told me that I wasn't making enough insulin and now you are telling me that I am making too much, which is it?"

When patients ask this question, it is clearly a case of not understanding insulin resistance. I have found there to be a great many people with diabetes, including some who have had it for many years, who don't understand the concept of insulin resistance. It is important to remember the time frame in which the actual events occur.

In the period of time prior to developing diabetes, when the patient becomes increasingly more insulin resistant and the doors to the cells fail to open as they should, the beta cells in the pancreas will, over time, increase the amount of insulin they produce. This in turn will fatigue the beta cells to the point that they will gradually cease to manufacture insulin. At this point insulin production will start to decline. This will continue as more beta cells become exhausted and quit working. In the development of type 2 diabetes, when insulin resistance is the cause, there is a progressive increase in insulin production above normal levels for a number of years followed by a decrease in insulin production to below normal levels.

Also, keep in mind that the time it takes to develop type 2 diabetes varies from person to person. Typically someone could be insulin resistant for five to ten years before becoming diabetic. In my example I indicated that the diabetes took about five years to develop, with the first sign of insulin resistance starting to show up in June of 2000 and the distinction of having diabetes not until June of 2005. It is possible for the first signs of insulin resistance to start showing up as early as ten years prior to actually becoming diabetic.

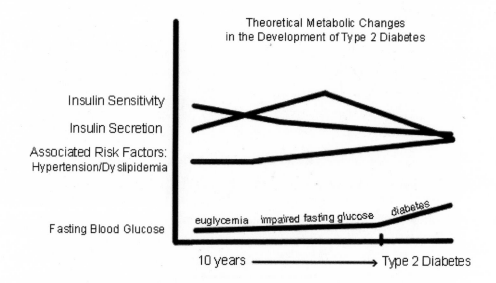

The relationship between insulin resistance and insulin sensitivity and how it can lead to the development of impaired glucose tolerance and type 2 diabetes over the course of approximately 10 years.

Rusty Hinges

By now you have probably already started wondering, "Why do the doors to the muscle, fat and liver cells become hard to open?" Rusty hinges. It's as if the hinges on the doors to the cells become rusty. With rusty hinges on the doors, the doors do not open as easily as they should, and it takes more insulin to get the doors open. Having rusty hinges is another way of describing insulin resistance. As an example, you may hear someone say, "Hey, guess what I heard about Betty at the beauty shop? Doris was telling me the doctor told her she had rusty hinges. He also told her she needed to start walking everyday." Or, "I had a check up with my doctor last week, and she said it looked as though I had gained a few pounds. When I told her it was more than a few, that I had gained almost 25 pounds in 6 months, she said that the weight gain had probably caused my hinges to start getting rusty."

Rarely, would anyone know that the hinges on the doors to their muscle, fat and liver cells are getting rusty because there are no physical symptoms associated with having rusty hinges, at least nothing most people would likely associate with this problem. After all, blood sugar levels remain normal as long as the beta cells continue to make all of the insulin necessary to get the doors to the cells open.

On the other hand, it is likely that most physicians and many other health care personnel could easily spot someone with rusty hinges just by looking at them or even by asking them several questions. Probably the biggest problem with not knowing that the hinges are rusty is that you don't do anything to try to fix them, and the rusty hinges continue to get worse. The worse they get the more insulin the beta cells have to make in order to get the doors to the cells open.

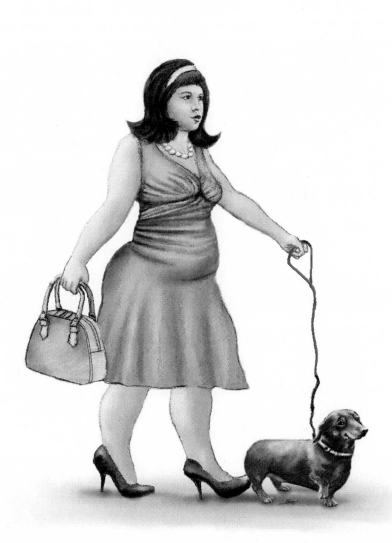

What insulin resistance or "rusty hinges" looks like.

I said exercise has the same effect as if you were to take sand paper and sand rust off the hinges and then spray the hinges with WD-40.

Now, in reality I think we would all agree that there are no doors with hinges on them inside our bodies. I mean really, think about it, it would be impossible to make hinges that small! But explaining the concept of insulin resistance using doors with rusty hinges and then how weight loss and exercise can improve insulin resistance as I do makes it easier to understand, at least it seems to, for most people. The truth is there is a lot of complex biochemistry that facilitates the entry of glucose into the various muscle, fat and liver cells throughout the body. Cell biologists and biochemists cannot say for sure why exercise makes it so much easier for glucose to enter the cells; they just know it does.

Although the whole story has yet to be figured out, at least we know the role exercise plays in lowering insulin resistance and how important it is to exercise. Eventually, I am confident researchers will figure out the rest of the story, and someday we will know exactly what happens at the cellular level and how exercise improves the ability of insulin to get glucose into the cell. Until that day and probably even after, I will talk about cell doors with rusty hinges when referring to insulin resistance and how performing exercise, in effect, is like sanding the rust off the hinges and spraying them with WD-40. At least in class it gets the point across.

Even if we knew the biochemistry of how exercise lowered insulin resistance, and even if we assumed that I understood all of the complex biochemistry involved, I very likely would never mention any of it in a class, as it would be very difficult to understand, that is unless you are a biochemist or cell biologist. Teaching at that level would be like speaking Spanish to a class of Japanese. The students probably wouldn't learn much.

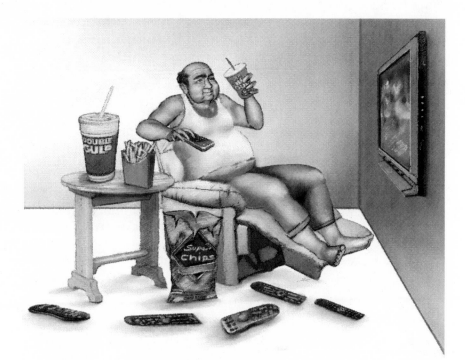

A classic example of rusty hinges in the making, too much fat and too little physical activity.

What Causes Rusty Hinges? In most cases, being overweight or obese and being inactive cause the rusty hinges. Actually, it is not so much being overweight as it is being over fat. What's the difference between being overweight and being over fat? There is a huge difference. Take a bodybuilder, for example. He may be 6 feet tall and weigh 230 pounds, but he is nearly solid muscle. The percentage of body fat is less than 5 percent. This is pretty typical of a professional body builder. According to normal standards this man would be overweight, and if you did not see him and only knew his height and weight, you would think he is over weight and, therefore, fat.

This is obviously not the case. It is not a health risk to be overweight if the extra weight is muscle. On the contrary, you may compare this body builder with another man that is 6 feet, 230 pounds and has a percentage of body fat that is 32 percent. This man would look considerably different from the body builder and would probably have a considerably bigger belly on him. This man would be considered overweight as well, but his increase in weight above normal levels would be attributed to carrying too much fat on his body. A more accurate description of this man would be over fat.

There are many people who are overweight, according to height and weight tables, that are not over fat and are, therefore, not insulin resistant and not at an increased risk for developing diabetes. These people are over weight because they possess a lot of muscle mass. There is no known health risk associated with that. Professional athletes and people who exercise a lot may build a lot of muscle mass and are a good example of this. Did you know that for every 2.2 kilograms you weigh above what is recommended for your height, you increase your risk of developing diabetes 4.5 percent? (2)

No one can say why being over fat and leading an inactive lifestyle causes "rusty hinges" or "insulin resistance"; we just know that it happens. I did an extensive review of the scientific literature looking for the biochemical basis of insulin resistance and how being over fat and getting too little exercise could have a causal relationship. It revealed nothing, at least not enough for me to be able to tell you what it is about not getting enough exercise and carrying excess body fat that causes insulin resistance.

Although a lot has been learned about insulin resistance over the last few years, we are not at a point of understanding why being over fat and sedentary causes the hinges on the doors to the muscle, fat and liver cells to become rusty; we just know that it does, and we make recommendations based on that. (3)

What we do know and is very clear is that insulin resistance is one of nearly a half dozen abnormalities that make up what is known as "the metabolic syndrome," a cluster of disorders that are frequently present when the diagnosis of diabetes is made. The metabolic syndrome has also been referred to as "Syndrome X" or "the deadly quartet."

Chapter 2
The Metabolic Syndrome

Anything that can be referred to as the "deadly quartet" is definitely something you want to stay away from. It's a scary name and rightfully so. Perhaps it earned its name due to the multiple and often serious or fatal medical problems that can result from having the "deadly quartet" or the more commonly used term, and the term I will use, "the metabolic syndrome."

The metabolic syndrome is a cluster of medical abnormalities that very often precedes the development of type 2 diabetes and significantly increases the risk for heart disease.

Dyslipidemia, high blood pressure, increased waist circumference and insulin resistance all make up what is known as the metabolic syndrome. Dyslipidemia is a medical term that is used when the amount of cholesterol and triglycerides in the blood are outside the normal range. When any of these levels are above normal, or below normal as in the case of high density cholesterol, it increases the likelihood of heart disease, and the more levels that are out of range, the greater the risk of developing heart disease.

As stated a moment ago, in many cases the metabolic syndrome ultimately leads to the development of type 2 diabetes and heart disease. It is interesting to note that the same lifestyle that typically leads to type 2 diabetes is what causes the metabolic syndrome, that being, well, you should know by now, being overweight and not getting enough exercise!

People often ask me if there are any signs or clues to alert them that they may be in the process of developing type 2 diabetes. One outstanding clue is if their doctor had ever diagnosed them as having the metabolic syndrome. For diagnosis a patient needs to have at least three out of the six or so components that make up the metabolic syndrome. A person may believe they are doing all right because they only possess one or two of the abnormalities or components that make up the metabolic syndrome, but if this person is inactive and has an expanding abdominal girth, they are not all right and it is probably only a short matter of time before they meet criteria for diagnosis.

Keep in mind, however, that not everyone with the metabolic syndrome will go on to develop type 2 diabetes. Remember, there must be some genetic malfunction present in addition to a lifestyle of inactivity and being over fat that causes diabetes. Insulin resistance is just one component of the metabolic syndrome, and it is likely that many if not all of the other components of the metabolic syndrome are present when the diabetes is first discovered. It is at the time a person first becomes insulin resistant and starts producing greater than normal quantities of insulin that the risk of heart disease starts to increase. As insulin resistance worsens over time and more and more insulin is manufactured and released into the blood, it is likely the risk of heart disease will increase even further.

Hyperinsulinemia, the term used for describing increased levels of insulin in the blood stream, when due to insulin resistance, is thought to have a causal effect in the development of heart disease. (3) Greater than normal amounts of insulin in the blood when there is no insulin resistance is not likely to contribute to heart disease. At one time it was believed that anytime a person was hyperinsulinemic the risk of heart disease increased. (3)

If someone is diagnosed as having the metabolic syndrome, has a genetic predisposition for diabetes, but still has normal blood sugars, it is probably only a matter of time before the blood sugar levels become elevated above normal values and diabetes is diagnosed.

Early Diagnosis

It is extremely important for you to know if you have some of the abnormalities that make up the metabolic syndrome and the earlier the better. Not only is the metabolic syndrome likely to cause diabetes, but it may lead to heart disease as well. Although there is no guarantee, making lifestyle changes once you are found to have the metabolic syndrome but prior to actually developing heart disease or diabetes may prevent you from ever getting either one of them! Research has shown that simply having insulin resistance, with hyperinsulinemia, as discussed above, independent of it being one of the components of the metabolic syndrome, increases the risk of developing heart disease.

Early detection of the metabolic syndrome is vital, but more importantly, doing something about it is even more critical. The longer you have the components of the syndrome, the greater the chance that heart disease and diabetes will become a reality. Work with your doctor to treat the syndrome early and treat it aggressively to avoid future consequences.

Some doctors seem to put more emphasis on having the metabolic syndrome than others and are more aggressive with its treatment. I can tell you that is the kind of doctor I would want. It is important to remember that one of the most frequent and biggest mistakes people make is to downplay the significance of having the metabolic syndrome, or even diabetes, particularly if early on they don't feel any different than usual. If you wait until you see the first signs of complications, the disease has likely already done considerable damage and reversal of the complications, even with good diabetes care, is not possible. No matter how well a person takes care of themselves after the onset of complications, retinopathy, which is damage to the retina, neuropathy, which is damage to the nervous system, and nephropathy, damage to the kidneys, cannot be reversed. It can be treated with medications, etc., but not reversed. This is why it is so very important to initiate steps to treat the metabolic syndrome immediately upon its diagnosis and effectively manage the diabetes as soon as you find out you have it. I simply cannot emphasize this enough.

Characteristics of Metabolic Syndrome

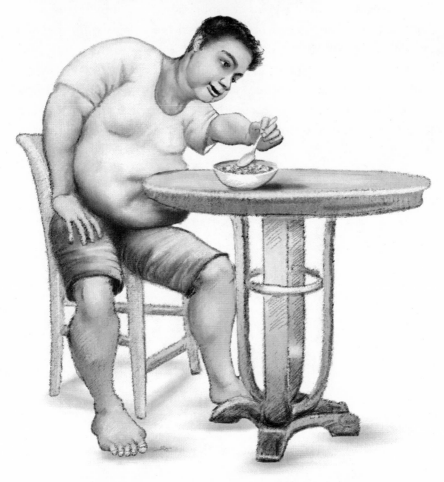

A waist circumference greater than 40 inches for a man is one
characteristic of the metabolic syndrome

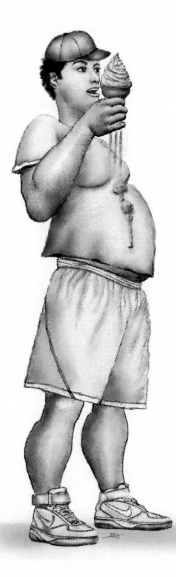

Eating too much of the wrong kind of foods is a major cause of the metabolic syndrome

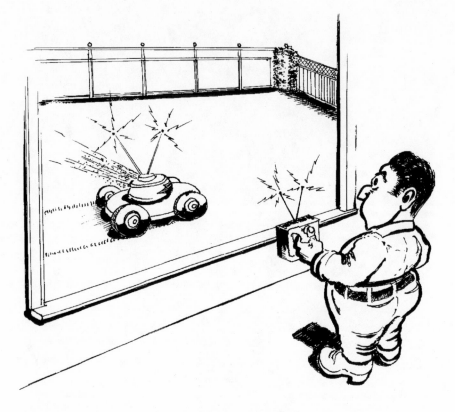

Avoiding exercise or physical activity is the other major cause of the metabolic syndrome.

If you carry excess fat around your waist, you are definitely at risk for having other abnormalities characteristic of the metabolic syndrome. This is known as being pear shaped. If in addition to that you get little to no regular exercise, you are at an even greater risk. Let's call those factors two strikes against you. If this sounds like you, it would be wise to get yourself to your doctor and let the doctor evaluate you thoroughly to see if you have the metabolic syndrome. If after the evaluation the doctor says that although overweight and inactive you have no other components of the metabolic syndrome, be happy, celebrate briefly, but don't get too happy; you are not out of the woods yet. You are lucky. You may not have the metabolic syndrome, now; however, it's just around the corner and just a matter of time before you do have it unless you make some lifestyle changes and quick. Remember, if you have one or more components of the metabolic syndrome already it will probably take some significant changes in your lifestyle to prevent having more of them in the near future.

Lifestyle

It is abundantly clear that leading a healthy lifestyle is the best way to avoid developing type 2 diabetes. If you are unfortunate enough to have already been diagnosed with type 2 diabetes, leading a healthy lifestyle is the best way to take care of it and reduce the risks of future diabetes related complications. Leading a healthy lifestyle means getting plenty of exercise, losing excess body fat if you have it, eating well balanced, nutritious, low fat meals and snacks, avoiding tobacco and keeping alcohol ingestion to a minimum.

Cigarette smoking is very dangerous for someone with type 2 diabetes and should be avoided at all costs. Similarly, excessive alcohol consumption can be particularly harmful for people with type 2 diabetes. For people with components of the metabolic syndrome or those that have the metabolic syndrome, and the approximately 57 million people that are pre-diabetic, without a doubt, the two most important things they can do is exercise regularly and reduce the amount of fat they are storing on their bodies. For men this probably means making the waistline smaller because this is where men tend to store extra body fat. For women this means making the hips and buttocks smaller as women tend to store extra fat in these areas.

Getting sufficient exercise on a regular basis and making wise food choices that reduce your caloric intake, slightly, over the long term, are your best bets to encourage fat loss. In fact, this method is really the only reasonable, effective and safe means for reducing excess fat and keeping it off. Additionally, making better food choices may have a profoundly positive effect on other components of the metabolic syndrome, such as your blood pressure and blood fats, commonly referred to as your lipid profile. Sometimes the inclusion of regular exercise and a more healthful diet into your lifestyle is all that is necessary to rid you of your metabolic syndrome. If so, that is great and maintaining this healthy way of living should significantly reduce your risk of developing heart disease, suffering a stroke, or being insulin resistant and subsequently developing type 2 diabetes.

Conversely, eating too much in general or eating foods high in fat or sugar or both certainly will cause weight gain and is likely to shoot the total cholesterol, LDL cholesterol and triglycerides, up and over desirable ranges. Eating like this is harmful enough; however, eating like this and leading a sedentary lifestyle at the same time can lead to disastrous consequences. Nothing healthy will result from a lifestyle like this.

For some people the incorporation of regular exercise and making better food choices is all it takes to normalize dyslipidemia (an abnormal lipid profile), blood pressure and decrease insulin resistance. Still others may need medication in addition to making positive lifestyle changes. In most all cases, however, the metabolic syndrome can be treated effectively. If all components of the metabolic syndrome are successfully treated, and in a timely manner, there is no reason why diabetes or heart disease should ever develop.

At the present time, however, two out of three people with diabetes die from heart disease every year. This causes me to wonder if the components that make up the metabolic syndrome are not being adequately controlled once diagnosed and continue to be minimized or ignored by a large majority of patients that have diabetes. Keep in mind that many of the components that are part of the metabolic syndrome are present for up to ten years prior to the actual onset of type 2 diabetes. Because of this, the increased risk of heart disease and stroke generally associated with the onset of diabetes actually begins with the diagnosis of the first component of the metabolic syndrome. Then as more components appear the risk increases. It is likely that by the time a patient's blood sugar level first rises above normal and he/she is diagnosed with type 2 diabetes, they already have some degree of heart disease. This is because the risk of developing problems with the heart, brain and circulatory system increases in a somewhat exponential fashion with each additional component of the metabolic syndrome.

It is entirely possible that one of the reasons two out of three people with type 2 diabetes die from heart disease or stroke is because they are focusing only on their blood glucose values and not their cardiovascular risk factors.

Prior to developing diabetes, someone's primary goal may have been to keep an eye on their cholesterol and triglyceride levels. Now with a new diagnosis of type 2 diabetes, they may shift their focus towards getting their hemoglobin A1C down to desirable levels and for the time being, pay less attention to controlling their cardiovascular risk factors. Doing that could be a very big and costly mistake. Hemoglobin A1C, usually seen written as HbA1C as I will refer to it throughout the rest of this book, is a blood test that indicates what blood glucose levels have been for the past three months. To a person with diabetes their HbA1C score is to them what a handicap is to a golfer. To someone who plays golf, knowing another golfer's handicap says a lot about the other golfer. It's a good way to find out just how good or not good the other player is. Similarly, a doctor or diabetes educator can quickly assess how well a patient has been able to control his or her blood glucose levels over the last 3-4 months simply by knowing their HbA1C score. The higher the score, the higher the blood glucose levels have been. The lower the score, the better the blood glucose levels have been.

A good comprehensive diabetes education program is going to stress the importance of both, controlling blood glucose levels, thereby keeping HbA1C scores down to reduce the risks of developing micro vascular complications, and controlling the cardiovascular risk factors, primarily responsible for causing macro vascular disease, that being heart disease and stroke.

One of the concepts I tend to really emphasize when teaching class is that it is just as important to control the cardiovascular risk factors mentioned above (blood pressure and lipid profile), as it is to control blood glucose levels.

I feel so strongly about this that the name I had chosen for this book originally was, "It's what's under the surface of the water that kills you." The majority of the cover was going to be an illustration of a big iceberg with only the tip of the iceberg protruding above the water. The iceberg was going to be in the foreground with a cruise ship seen in the far distance. The calm water could be seen reflecting moonlight back up into the sky. I was even going to add a few shiny stars in addition to a nearly full moon. What I hadn't decided on yet was how to make the part of the iceberg under the water look ominous. When I draw this picture on the board in class, I point to the part of the iceberg above water and ask someone in class what we call this part of the iceberg. Usually it only takes a few guesses before someone shouts the correct answer, "It's the tip of the iceberg."

I then ask one or more of the patients if they know exactly what is wrong with them or how did the doctor discover you had diabetes. Regardless of which question I ask, the answer is usually about the same. "I have too much sugar in my blood," or, "The doctor said the blood test showed there was too much sugar in my blood." I then turn to the board, and in the little area of the iceberg above the water I write, "the tip of the ice berg." I then draw an upward arrow and the letters BS, indicating increased blood sugar. I then tell the class that having too much sugar in the blood is the tip of the iceberg when it comes to having type 2 diabetes. There is a whole lot more to having diabetes than having too much sugar in the blood. Type 2 Diabetes is a cluster of metabolic disorders, and elevated blood sugar levels is just one of them. To successfully control type 2 diabetes all of the metabolic disorders must be controlled.

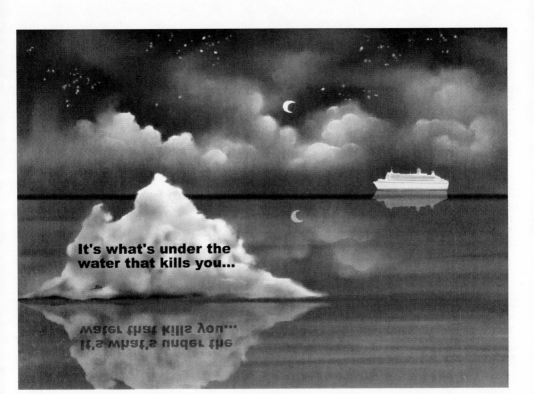

At this point, in the area under the tip of the iceberg, and under the surface of the water, I list the rest of the metabolic disorders usually accompanying elevated blood sugar levels; high blood pressure, elevated total cholesterol and LDL cholesterol, decreased HDL cholesterol and above normal triglycerides. When I turn to face the class after writing this on the board I frequently notice one or more of the patients nodding their head and grinning. "Why are you nodding and grinning," I ask? They point to the board and tell me, "That's me. You're talking about me. I have every one of those problems."

Others ask if they are destined to develop the other metabolic disorders if they don't have them yet. I tell them it is not a certainty, however, there is a much greater likelihood they will develop them because they already have elevated blood sugar levels.

This news that there is more to diabetes than having too much sugar in the blood comes as a shock to a lot of class participants. This is information they have never heard before.

I sometimes will stop teaching for a minute and ask the class a few questions. "How many of you know what your social security number is? If you have a cell phone, do you know your cell phone number? If you have a computer do you remember your password to log on? How about your street address?" It probably comes as no surprise to you that almost without fail, class participants know all of these answers. I then congratulate them on a job well done, so far, and tell them I have just a few more questions.

"What is your total cholesterol level and do you know what it should be? How about your LDL cholesterol, do you know what it is? Do you know what it should be? One more, how about your triglycerides? Do you know what is considered normal?

Unfortunately, most of my patients knew the answers to the early questions but did a very poor job with the questions regarding their blood fats.

I then ask them which of the answers they don't know are the most important to know. Obviously, you need to know your social security number and cell phone number, etc., and you have made a point to do so. Have you made the same effort to know the levels of your various blood fats and the recommendations as to what they should be? I can sadly report that most people don't know their most recent lab values and those who do often do not know the desirable range.

Doctor's are now frequently recommending that their diabetes patients, because of their increased risk for developing heart disease or having a stroke, adhere to a more strict set of blood lipid guidelines than is routinely recommended for people without diabetes.

When your doctor tells you that your blood work looks good, do you know which guidelines he or she is following? Do you think you should? Maybe your lab work looks good based on the less strict guidelines usually referred to as the "desirable range" found on most lab results sheets but would not be considered acceptable based on the more strict guidelines many physicians are now following for their patients with diabetes.

I suggest to patients that they ask for a copy of their lab work before leaving the doctor's office. If reading or understanding the result sheet is difficult, I suggest that you ask someone at the doctor's office to help you. You need to know where you stand. Is your cholesterol above the recommended level and maybe your triglycerides too? If so, what is your doctor doing to address this? I am hopeful that one of the benefits you will gain from reading this book is that you will become better informed about diabetes and capable of taking more responsibility in the treatment of the disease.

I never want anyone to walk out of my classes feeling hopeless. I'm concerned that sometimes patients with many or all of the lipid abnormalities and high blood pressure may feel this way, like they have so many things wrong with them that there is no point in even trying to get better.

On the contrary, these patients just have a lot more room for improvement. Do you remember ever being asked the question, "If a tree fell in the forest but there was no one there to hear it, would it make any noise?" Similarly, if you have been diagnosed as having high blood pressure but now take medicine to bring your blood pressure down to normal levels, do you still have high blood pressure? Well, yes, you do have high blood pressure but in reality you don't. And if that last sentence doesn't make things crystal clear, try this: For the purposes of filling out medical forms, questionnaires and applying for life insurance, yes, you are hypertensive, you have high blood pressure. However, if your high blood pressure is treated effectively, then it is normal.

The same can be said for cholesterol and triglyceride levels. If a medication or combination of medications is taken that corrects these abnormalities, do you still have dyslipidemia, abnormal levels of fat in the blood? You could say yes, you have dyslipidemia, but it is controlled or corrected with medication, or yes, you are hypertensive, but it is well controlled with medication and lifestyle modifications, if that is the case. It is entirely possible to possess all of the major cardiovascular risk factors for heart disease and stroke, however, with the help of prescription medications, exercise, and by making better food choices bring every risk factor back into normal range. If this were to happen, the risk of having a heart attack or stroke would drop dramatically.

I have had patients show me the results of their latest lab work and I become envious. Their lab work looks great, far better than mine. That is not to say mine is bad, but I like theirs better. These are patients previously diagnosed with dyslipidemia who now, with the inclusion of exercise, better nutrition and medication, or some combination of these three treatments, have far better than average lipid values. During the seven years that I worked with patients in our diabetes exercise facility, I observed that the patients with the very best lipid profiles took a cholesterol or triglyceride lowering medication. My point here being that even if every metabolic disorder commonly associated with diabetes were present in a patient, there are an abundance of medications and strategies available to successfully treat the disorder, thereby reducing the risk of heart disease and stroke.

As for the micro vascular complications, those being eye, nerve and kidney disease, it is imperative to keep the HbA1C score as low as possible and definitely below 7 percent. A very large and frequently referred to study known as the DCCT (The Diabetes Control and Complications Trial), completed in the late 1990's, showed that diabetes patients able to maintain very tight or good control of their blood glucose levels, demonstrated by a hemoglobin A1C of less than 7 percent, had significantly fewer micro vascular complications. (4) The American Diabetes Association recommends a score of less than 7 percent, which correlates to average blood glucose values of approximately 170mg/dl. (5)

Table 1 - Correlation between HbA1C level and mean plasma glucose levels on multiple testing over 2-3 months

Hemoglobin A1C (HbA1C)	Average Blood Glucose (Mg/dl)
13.0%	380
12.0%	345
11.0%	310
10.0%	275
9.0%	240
8.0%	205
7.0%	170
6.0%	135
5.0%	100

At this point in class I like to summarize the point I have been trying to make with the following equation:

Figure 1

$$\underline{HbA1C < 7\%} + \underline{Controlling\ cardiovascular\ risk\ factors} = \underline{Good\ health}$$

| 50% | 50% | 100% |

For the best chances of maintaining good health when you have type 2 diabetes, HbA1C scores need to be maintained below 7 percent and cardiovascular risk factors need to be well controlled. It is simply not enough, or only half the battle, to control one without the other.

Alternative Theories about Decreased Insulin Production

Before going any further I want to acknowledge that not everyone agrees as to what specifically causes insulin production to drop and what causes a decline in the number of functioning beta cells in patients who have developed type 2 diabetes.

When you read about diabetes in publications such as *Diabetes Forecast, Diabetes Health, Diabetes Self- Management* or *The Diabetes Educator,* you will find that almost universally they will state that in most cases the cause of type 2 diabetes is the inability of the beta cells of the pancreas to make adequate amounts of insulin (insufficient insulin production), and the inability of the body's cells to utilize the insulin as it should (insulin resistance). These facts are not disputed. As for why insulin production drops and why there seems to be a gradual decline in the number of functioning beta cells, there is not universal agreement.

In the next several pages I will share some of the more recent theories of how type 2 diabetes is developed.

It has always been felt that genetics played a strong role in the development of type 2 diabetes but there is uncertainty as to how significant a role that was. When I am interviewing newly diagnosed type 2 diabetes patients, they will frequently tell me that their mom or dad has diabetes and that they got it from them. The inference seems to be that they were destined to develop diabetes because of the genetic influence passed on to them by their mom or dad, or both.

Patients need to understand that having a mom or dad with diabetes will make it easier for them to develop diabetes but does not guarantee they will get it. Having a parent, or parents, with diabetes just improves the conditions or increases the odds for developing diabetes. People unfortunate enough to have a family history of diabetes need to work extra hard at keeping their bodyweight normal and getting plenty of daily exercise.

Some people with a strong family history of diabetes may develop the disease no matter what efforts they make to avoid it, while others are able to sidestep diabetes altogether by leading a very active and healthy lifestyle. Although insulin resistance, caused by inactivity or being overweight or obese leads to type 2 diabetes about 80 percent of the time, an underlying genetic predisposition is thought to be necessary in order to develop diabetes. This theory would help explain why everyone that is overweight and inactive does not have diabetes.

As for the twenty percent of patients with type 2 diabetes who did not develop it this way, there are other causes. These causes may include medication induced diabetes and diabetes that results secondary to another medical condition. These cases make up by far the minority of patients with type 2 diabetes. I don't want to elaborate more than that on these cases as it is beyond the focus of his book.

For those of you either needing or wanting a little refresher concerning genetics, the next several paragraphs are for you. If, on the other hand, you find learning about genes and genetics is dull and feel it unnecessary, please feel free to skip down several paragraphs and pick up the explanation there, you won't be hurting my feelings.

You have undoubtedly heard the saying that no two people are exactly alike. No two people are exactly alike because inside each of us, in every cell of our bodies, is a set of instructions indicating what we are to be like. Every cell, whether it is a cell in our thumb or a cell in our knee, has a complete set of instructions or blueprint as to how we are put together and how our bodies are supposed to work. These instructions are on strands of what we call DNA, deoxyribonucleic acid. Each strand of DNA contains a multitude of genes. A gene is a particular section of the DNA strand where instructions for a particular body function reside. (6)

On both sides of this gene are genes that are responsible for other parts of the body. You can imagine what a tremendous amount of information there must be on a single strand of DNA. Also amazing is how all of the information on the DNA strands has to fit into each little cell of our body. This is possible because the DNA strands arrange themselves in a twisted ladder formation referred to as a "double helix". This double helix then wraps itself around some proteins and pack together to form a chromosome.

There are 46 chromosomes in each human cell. Twenty-three of the chromosomes or literally half the genetic information comes from the mom with the other 23 chromosomes coming from the dad. With genetic information coming from both parents, you can see why kids resemble their mom in some ways and their dad in other ways.

Researchers are looking at gene mutations, or mutations involving several genes, that may be responsible for making conditions ripe so that when combined with sedentary lifestyle and being overweight, diabetes occurs. As an example, a mutation of a gene involved in the manufacture of enzymes used in fat metabolism or genes involved in the location of fat storage may be all that is necessary from a genetic standpoint to encourage the development of diabetes. At present, it is still not clear as to which genetic abnormalities or how many genetic abnormalities are factors in developing diabetes.

Research conducted over the last 30 years by the NIDDK with the help of the Pima Indians has helped prove that overweight and/or obesity is a major risk factor in the development of type 2 diabetes. (7) This tribe of Pimas, living in Arizona and Mexico, has an extremely high incidence of type 2 diabetes. Coincidentally, they are also known to have a high percentage of overweight and obesity people as well. The NIDDK reports that one-half of adult Pima Indians have diabetes and that 95 percent of those with diabetes are overweight. Prior to World War II, however, the Pima Indians were not significantly different in their bodyweight from other tribes of Indians, indicating that it has not always been this way. One interesting discovery the NIDDK found when studying the Pima tribe was that before gaining weight, overweight people have a slower metabolic rate when compared to people of the same weight. This fact coupled with a heavy consumption of fats and genetic predisposition to store excess fat, may have been what led to the epidemic proportions of overweight people in this tribe.

One theory proposed back in 1962 by geneticist James Neel, was that a "thrifty gene" may have helped the Pimas become overweight. (7) Neel theorized that the Pimas experienced periods when food was plentiful, as when the hunting and fishing were good, and times when food was scarce. To survive during times of famine, Neel suggested that the Pimas developed a "thrifty" gene that allowed them to store fat when food was abundant that they could later use when food was scarce. The so-called "thrifty" gene worked well for the tribe under these conditions; but later when obtaining food was not a problem and with less physical activity, the gene worked to their detriment. The result being half the tribe now having type 2 diabetes of which 95 percent are overweight or obese.

Dr. Eric Ravussin, a visiting scientist at the Phoenix Epidemiology and Clinical Research Branch at NIDDK, has studied the Pima Indians since 1984 and agrees with the thrifty gene theory, at least in the case of the Pima Indians. Dr. Ravussin recently found a tribe of Pimas in Mexico still living as their ancestors had lived many years ago. Out of 35 Mexican Pima Indians studied, only three had diabetes and the majority of the tribe was not overweight. (7) This is quite a contrast to the Pima tribe in Arizona.

At a professional conference I attended in June of 2006 I had the pleasure of eating breakfast with Dr. Boyd Eaton, a radiologist and medical anthropologist from Emory University and proclaimed "evolutionary nutrition" expert by *USA Weekend*. Dr. Eaton is the author of several books including,

The Paleolithic Prescription: A program of Diet and Exercise and a Design for Living.

As it turned out Dr. Eaton was to be a presenter at the conference later that day. When Dr. Eaton asked what I did for a living and learned of my profession as a diabetes educator, our conversation soon focused on what I learned was a passion of his, the contrast between our modern day diet and associated health problems, (including insulin resistance and diabetes) and the lifestyle and health of our ancestors thousands of years ago.

During our conversation and later in his presentation, he told me that there is more of a genetic difference between an African American and Caucasian than between modern man and man thousands of years ago. In fact, and I quote, " 99.9 percent of our genetic heritage dates from about 40,000 years ago-before our biological ancestors had even evolved into Homo Sapiens-and that 99.99 percent of our genes were formed prior to the development of agriculture some 10,000 years ago. That the vast majority of our genes are ancient in origin means that nearly all of our biochemistry and physiology are fine-tuned to conditions of life that existed before 10,000 years ago. Genetically, our bodies are now virtually the same as they were then. The problem is, our diet isn't."

Could this be the cause of our diabetes? Dr. Eaton goes on to say, "10,000 years ago, pre-agriculture , we were all hunter-gatherers, hunting meat such as deer and bison, gathering fruits, vegetables and nuts. It was a lifestyle that required considerable physical exertion. Skeletal remains indicate that our ancestors were typically more muscular than we are today." With few exceptions, we now live in a time that requires very little physical exertion. After all, when was the last time you had to hunt down and kill your breakfast? Could this be the cause of our diabetes? Could it be a combination of both our lifestyle, in general, what we eat, and what we do, or don't do, causing us to be out of sync with our genes?

Dr. Eaton believes that a dramatic shift away from eating as our ancestors did is responsible for 'diseases of civilization" now accounting for 75 percent of all deaths in the West. (8)

It appears that whether it is a gene mutation that affects the way fat is metabolized, or utilizing less calories than consumed, or an inability to restrict excessive eating that leads to obesity, being overweight or obese and leading a sedentary lifestyle are the greatest controllable, causative factors in the development of type 2 diabetes. In the event you missed what I just stated I will state it again, it's that important! Being overweight or obese and leading a sedentary lifestyle are the greatest controllable, causative factors in the development of type 2 diabetes. As the incidence of overweight and obesity steadily increases and the decline in physical activity and exercise continues, researchers look for their causes and search for solutions that will turn these trends around. Type 2 diabetes, once called "adult onset" or even sometimes unofficially referred to as "old age" diabetes is now referred to as "a lifestyle" illness. The term "adult onset" had to be changed, as it is no longer descriptive of so many now being diagnosed.

Today, teenagers in general, are less physically active than ever before, leading to more cases of insulin resistance and ultimately to type 2 diabetes for those unfortunate enough to be genetically predisposed. Fifteen years ago it was extremely rare to have someone in class that was under fifty years old; today it is commonplace.

From the information available on type 2 diabetes today, the general consensus is that even considering genetic influences, in most cases, a person's lifestyle habits are the best indicator of their tendency to develop type 2 diabetes.

Preventing Type 2 Diabetes, in a Nutshell

Do more of this:	And less of this:
Push the lawn mower	Using a riding lawnmower
Rake the leaves	Using a blower
Wash the car yourself	Going through the car wash
Lift and close the garage door	Using the remote door opener
Get up to change the TV channel	Changing channels with the remote
Crank the pencil sharpener	Using an electric pencil sharpener
Hang the laundry	Using a clothes dryer

Try to look more like this:	And less like this:
Slender and firm	Large and soft

Eat more of this:	And less of this:
Lean cuts of meat, fish and vegetables	High carbohydrate and high fat foods

After the Diagnosis

So now what do you do? You have just been told you have diabetes. This usually comes as quite a shock to most people, although there are many who say they were expecting it because of their strong family history. Without a doubt, being told you have diabetes is life altering. From that moment forward it is unlikely those diagnosed will eat many meals without consciously or subconsciously wondering what the effect on their blood glucose level will be. Those people who have always enjoyed good health and have had few if any health problems may be taken back the most. Anger, resentment, denial, depression, and a sense of loss, are all very common feelings people experience. Displays of anger, denial or resentment early on are common and have little bearing on a patient's ability to successfully take care of the diabetes long term.

Problems do arise when a patient's anger or depression, as an example, keep the patient from doing what is necessary to care for the disease. I have seen many patients who have been in denial of the diabetes for months to sometimes a year or more, this in spite of the fact that the patient is already experiencing one or more complications from the disease and has laboratory values that clearly indicate diabetes. Particularly sad and frustrating is when this situation involves a young person and a lack of proper care early after diagnosis leads to a lifetime of living with complications. It is reasonable to argue that when blood glucose levels are only slightly elevated above normal values, the less critical it is for the patient to make immediate and drastic changes in lifestyle. Conversely, when a patient is found to have a high HbA1C, it is extremely important that the patient accepts the illness and begins treating it aggressively. Every effort should be made to lower high blood glucose levels to desirable ranges as quickly as possible to reduce the risk of complications to the eyes, nerves and kidneys.

After Acceptance

Imagine being the captain of a ship and sailing the seas without a compass or stars to guide you. Imagine being a contractor and building a skyscraper with no blueprints.

Imagine being diabetic and taking good care of your diabetes without instruction. The fact is, it is no more likely you can manage your diabetes without instruction than the builder can build a building without blueprints or the captain can steer a ship without a compass or stars to guide him. Still, millions of people try to take care of their diabetes with no formal instruction.

"I know what I need to do, I don't need to go to some diabetes class for that, I just got to back off on my sweets," is the feeling of many.

"I know why I got this. I've just been eating too much the last couple of months and I got to just start watching it and I will be alright," is another common attitude.

Unfortunately, there are too many patients who mistakenly believe it is all about food, what you eat and don't eat. These patients may be motivated to attend a nutrition class or see a dietician one on one, but they are resistant to consider a comprehensive diabetes class, feeling it is unnecessary.

Patients need to be told early on, probably at the time of diagnosis, that to successfully manage type 2 diabetes, comprehensive diabetes education is a must. Formal instruction provided by a certified diabetes educator is usually a covered benefit and is definitely the way to go. For patients without health insurance, formal instruction is still the way to go; however, it may be a little more difficult to find.

Public hospitals sometimes offer free diabetes classes. The American Diabetes Association and American Association of Diabetes Educators both have web sites and would be a good place to start looking for what free education may be available in your area. The ADA and AADE websites are also loaded with information you may find useful. If formal education is not feasible, then I would recommend getting books from the library and reading all you can about diabetes. Look for health fairs at local hospitals or malls where you could talk with a diabetes educator or dietitian to answer questions not answered in books.

Misinformation: Don't believe everything you hear or read about diabetes, that is, unless it was me who said it or wrote it.

A few words of caution: be wary of people you meet who have had diabetes for a long time and want to tell you how to take care of it. They mean well and are probably genuinely trying to help you; however, their good intentions may backfire if the information that they give you is wrong. In fact, I prefer that newly diagnosed patients pretty much discount what veteran patients tell them regarding treatment. The veteran patient with long standing diabetes may not have had an education update in 5-10 years and may pass on outdated or inaccurate information to the new patient. This might be the lady down the street who tells you she figured out that she could eat pretty much whatever she wants as long as she adjusts how much insulin she takes each day. This is really bad advice and certainly something we don't want new patients to listen to.

I think many times these veterans of the disease start to believe they must know all there is to know about it because they have lived with it for so long. In reality there is probably a lot of new treatment information they know nothing about. When I teach a class that has a mixture of newly diagnosed patients and patients who have had diabetes for many years, I tell the patients with the longstanding history to take everything they know about diabetes and shove it to one side of their head, leaving room in the other side for new information they may have never heard before.

I have found that sometimes patients who have had diabetes for many years are resistant to new methods of treating the disease and it takes a lot of effort to convince them they would probably be better off with a new treatment regimen. I also tell them that if it has been longer than five years since the last time they attended a formal diabetes education class, they are due for a refresher. There is a lot of new information out there they need to know about, information that very likely will improve their ability to control their diabetes.

Chapter 3
Diagnosing Diabetes

There are several ways diabetes can be diagnosed. The approach I will summarize here is based on the most recent national guidelines established by the American Diabetes Association. (9)

When you first wake up in the morning, before you eat or drink anything, assuming you did not get up and eat or drink during the night after going to bed, you are in what is called a "fasting state." Fasting can be defined as no caloric intake for at least 8 hours. While in a fasting state your blood glucose levels should be below 100mg/dl. This means that for every deciliter of blood, which is slightly less than ½ cup, in your body, there should be less than 100 milligrams of sugar. A fasting blood glucose level above 100mg/dl. is abnormal. Two fasting readings above 100mg/dl. but less than 126mg/dl. indicate you have what is referred to as "Impaired fasting glucose" and are probably on your way to developing diabetes. In fact, impaired fasting glucose is also commonly referred to as pre-diabetes.

If two fasting blood glucose levels are above 126mg/dl., you meet the criteria for having diabetes, particularly if you are exhibiting symptoms such as fatigue, extreme thirst, frequent urination, changes in vision, and possibly unexplained weight loss. Your physician is really the only one who can ultimately make the diagnosis, and if you suspect that you have diabetes, you should consult your physician.

Diabetes can also be diagnosed based on the results of two random blood glucose readings. Random blood glucose is any blood glucose test that is performed when you are not in the fasting state. This could be right after a meal or mid afternoon. Random blood glucose readings in excess of 200mg/dl., on two occasions also indicate diabetes.

Still a third method of identifying diabetes is by having a glucose tolerance test. This test involves drinking a prescribed quantity of a glucose solution and then having your blood glucose levels checked at periodic intervals to see how much and how quickly the blood glucose levels come back down. This test is not usually considered necessary for the diagnosis to be made; however, it is sometimes still utilized.

Table 2 - Criteria for the Diagnosis of Diabetes

1. Symptoms of diabetes and a casual plasma glucose $\geq$ 200 mg/dl. (11.1 mmol/l). Casual is defined as any time of day without regard to time since last meal. The classic symptoms of diabetes include polyuria, polydipsia, and unexplained weight loss.

OR

2. Fasting plasma glucose (FPG) $\geq$ 126mg/dl. (7.0mmol/l). Fasting is defined as no caloric intake for at least 8 hours.

OR

3. 2-hour plasma glucose $\geq$ 200 mg/dl. (11.1mmol/l) during an Oral Glucose Tolerance Test.

The test should be performed as described by the World Health Organization, using a glucose load containing the equivalent of 75-g anyhydrous glucose dissolved in water.

Borderline Diabetes or a "Touch of Sugar"

So what do you have if your fasting blood glucose is above 100mg/dl., but below 126mg/dl.?

Until recently many health professionals called this "borderline diabetes." This phrase proved to be problematic because patients would leave the doctor's office after being told they were "borderline" but with little to no instruction as to what that meant or what to do about it. There was nothing about being told they were borderline that caused the patients to take this seriously.

Whether or not this had any influence on patients referring to their condition as simply "having a touch of sugar" is still anyone's guess. I have always considered this statement on par with calling a cardiac arrest "a little heart trouble." Several terms have been used to describe fasting blood glucose levels between 100mg/dl and 125mg/dl. These include, "impaired fasting glucose," "impaired glucose tolerance" and "pre-diabetes," terms that more accurately describe the situation.

In most cases, pre-diabetes will progress to type 2 diabetes unless of course the patient makes some immediate lifestyle changes. Patients diagnosed as having pre-diabetes who take it seriously and are willing to make some immediate lifestyle adjustments may sidestep ever developing diabetes by increasing exercise, reducing body fat and eating more carefully. It is likely that the sooner these lifestyle changes are implemented, the less likely diabetes will ever develop.

Unfortunately, most people don't understand the relationship between pre-diabetes and diabetes, and, therefore, don't take their pre-diabetes seriously. They put off or avoid diabetes education, altogether, continuing to lead a sedentary lifestyle, failing to lose weight and eating carelessly. For these people it's just a matter of time before their fasting blood glucose readings climb above 125mg/dl. and they too have diabetes.

Although no one can say how long it will take to progress from having pre-diabetes to diabetes, and the time frame probably varies from one person to another, it probably takes less time than most people think. This is particularly true for the person who exercises little, eats too much and is overweight. I have had patients come to class before, complaining of tingling and burning in their feet as well as vision disturbances, claiming to only have borderline diabetes or a "touch of sugar." That may have been the case a long time ago, but the truth is that they probably have had full-blown diabetes for quite a while now as evidenced by the tingling and burning in their feet, known as neuropathy, and vision problems, known as retinopathy. Pre-diabetes usually ends up being only a transition state patients pass through when going from normal blood glucose levels to high blood glucose levels and it does not last indefinitely.

Blood Glucose Guidelines

Blood glucose levels fluctuate throughout the day. This happens whether you have diabetes or not. However, people without diabetes do not fluctuate to near the extreme that many patients with diabetes might. Those without diabetes, even in extreme situations, may only fluctuate from a low of about 60mg/dl. early in the morning before breakfast, to a high after a meal of about 130mg/dl. or so. There are safeguard mechanisms inside the body that maintain blood glucose levels within fairly narrow limits whether in a fasting state, fed state, during exercise, or even after exhaustive exercise. So in the case of the non-diabetic person, even after exhaustive exercise lasting two or more hours, blood sugar levels in the blood may only drop to a low of 70-80mg/dl. and after two Thanksgiving dinners will probably not climb above 120-130mg/dl. This is a direct result of regulatory mechanisms in the body that are constantly working and making adjustments behind the scenes to maintain blood glucose levels in normal ranges, even under extreme conditions.

For the person with diabetes, the goals are virtually the same, to maintain normal or near normal blood glucose levels under all conditions; however, accomplishing this requires conscious effort and a serious commitment by the patient.

The American Diabetes Association recommends the following blood glucose guidelines for people with diabetes: (10)

Pre-meal blood glucose levels should be maintained between 90-130mg/dl. (10) This includes fasting levels first thing in the morning. Remember, fasting can be defined as 8 hours without caloric intake. And peak blood glucose levels after meals should be less than 180mg/dl. (10) Keep in mind that although these blood glucose goals are recommended for patients with diabetes, they are somewhat higher values than for someone without diabetes. Someone without diabetes is not likely to see numbers as high as 180mg/dl. after a meal and would see numbers a good bit lower than 130mg/dl. pre-meal.

A hemoglobin A1C blood test should be performed every three to six months. The score on this test should be less than 7 percent. A score of 7 percent correlates with an average blood glucose value of 170mg/dl. As a general rule for every 1 percent change in hemoglobin A1C, either up or down, the blood glucose value will change by 35 points. Exactly how this test works will be discussed in the upcoming section, blood glucose monitoring.

Blood glucose goals have changed somewhat over the years. New information now available as a result of more recent research indicates that maintaining even lower blood glucose levels is necessary to reduce the risk of what is referred to as "micro vascular disease." These complications are the result of small blood vessel damage. The retinopathy and neuropathy that I have previously mentioned are micro vascular complications. Micro vascular damage may also occur in the small vessels of the brain and kidneys.

When high blood sugar levels damage the small blood vessels of the kidney, it is called "nephropathy." This occurs when the kidneys are not able to filter the blood as they should, resulting in the accumulation of various harmful substances in the bloodstream. In many cases this eventually leads to total kidney failure and the necessity for kidney dialysis.

As it turns out diabetes is one of the leading causes of dialysis. Patients often find that the inability to adequately control their blood glucose levels results in a fairly rapid onset of retinopathy and neuropathy, whereas the onset of nephropathy may seem to develop more slowly. It is important to keep in mind, however, that every situation is different and it is impossible to predict a timeline as to when diabetes complications will occur. As new research teaches us more about what we need to do to improve the lives of people with diabetes, you may see these guidelines revised again. It is essential that patients stay up to date regarding any new recommendations as they are always made for the benefit of the patient.

The guidelines just mentioned were established by the American Diabetes Association and are current as of 2006.

Table 3 - Summary of Recommendations for Adults with Diabetes

Glycemic control:

HbA1C	<7.0 %*
Preprandial capillary plasma glucose	90-130mg/dl (5.0-7.2mmol/l)
Peak postprandial capillary plasma glucose[t]	<180mg/dl (10.0 mmol/l)
Blood Pressure	<130/80 mmHg

Key concepts in setting glycemic goals:

- A1C is the primary target for glycemic control
- Goals should be individualized
- Certain populations (children, pregnant women, and elderly) require special considerations
- More stringent glycemic goals (i.e., a normal A1C, < 6%) may

further reduce complications at the cost of increased risk of hypoglycemia

♦ Less intensive glycemic goals may be indicated in patients with severe or frequent hypoglycemia

♦ Postprandial glucose may be targeted if A1C goals are not met despite reaching preprandial glucose goals

---

*Referenced to a nondiabetic range of 4.0-6.0% using a DCCT-based assay. † Postprandial glucose measurements should be made 1-2 h after the beginning of the meal, generally peak levels in patients with diabetes.

Blood Glucose Monitoring

Self Blood Glucose monitoring is an effective way to see if what you are doing to control your diabetes is working. I recommend that all patients with diabetes check their blood glucose levels on a regular basis with few exceptions. To keep you from wondering the whole time you read this section if you are one of the few exceptions, I will go ahead and identify those who may not need to test their blood glucose levels regularly.

Patients at a very advanced age, who acquire diabetes but who seem to only have mildly elevated blood glucose levels and patients who are terminally ill and not expected to live much longer do not need to regularly check their blood glucose levels. That's about it. Pretty much everybody else should check his or her blood glucose levels at least several times a week to get some idea of his or her blood glucose levels.

Why am I not concerned with those two groups checking their blood glucose levels? Because long-term complications develop over the long term, and since the people in those two groups have circumstances that may prevent them from living long term, intensive management of their diabetes may not be appropriate in most cases. I guess you could say that I am not as concerned if someone in their eighties chooses not to check their blood glucose levels as someone in their forties. The younger you are the more time you have remaining in your life to develop complications, and so, the more I stress regular and frequent monitoring.

There are different opinions on this and recommendations on how often to test will vary from doctor to doctor. There is also no right time or wrong time to test blood glucose levels; however, the effectiveness of your treatment regimen may be easier to determine when blood glucose levels are checked at more specific times of the day. Ultimately, you should test your blood glucose levels frequently enough to get a good idea as to what your blood glucose patterns are throughout the day.

Hemoglobin A1C

Before recommending to patients how often to test their blood glucose, I ask them the value of their most recent hemoglobin A1C score, and I usually make my recommendations based largely on that. I do realize and keep in mind, however, that there are other factors to consider besides the HbA1C score, such as the availability of testing supplies, motivation, changes in treatment regimens and the fact that everyone may not be able or willing to test as often as I suggest.

The HbA1C is a blood test that tells you how well your blood glucose levels have been controlled over the last two to three months, and it is probably the best predictor of your risk for developing microvascular complications. This test is frequently performed four times per year. This is the way the test works. Inside every red blood cell there is a substance called hemoglobin. Hemoglobin is necessary for the delivery of oxygen to the millions of cells through out the body. Glucose in the blood enters the red blood cells much the same way it does other cells throughout the body. When the glucose enters the red blood cell it attaches itself, or sticks to the hemoglobin portion of the cell. This process is called glycosylation. The more glucose attached to the hemoglobin the greater the degree of glycosylation and the higher the hemoglobin A1C score. The less glucose attached to the hemoglobin the lower the degree of glycosylation and the lower the hemoglobin A1C score.The score you get on this test is similar to a grade your child may get on their report card.

Just as the grade on the report card tells you how well your child performed over the last semester in school, the HbA1C tells you how well you have been able to control your blood glucose levels over the last three to four months. Although fasting blood glucose readings may be ideal and lead you to believe your diabetes is in good control, your post lunch and dinner readings may be a bit high. If you are under the impression that your diabetes is in good control based solely on your fasting values, the HbA1C can be a real help in letting you know that things aren't necessarily as they seem. The HbA1C score will reflect not only your ideal fasting blood glucose readings but also the high readings after meals. Many patients that test only once per day before breakfast are quite surprised to see unexpectedly high HbA1C results reflecting post meal blood glucose levels. Seeing these results can motivate the patient to start testing blood glucose levels more frequently, including post meals. It is usually recommended to have an HbA1C test performed every three to six months.

Maintaining HbA1C scores below 7 percent is highly recommended, as it will significantly reduce your risk of developing the micro vascular complications. Conversely, if your score is higher then 7 percent, the likelihood of you developing those same complications rises significantly. This was shown quite clearly in the Diabetes Control and Complications Trial, the first study to show a link between higher HbA1C scores and an increase in micro vascular complications. (4) The higher the score and the longer it remains elevated, the greater the risk that someday, maybe sooner then you think, you will begin to experience some of the devastating complications associated with poor glucose control. It is therefore very important, as mentioned earlier in this book, on more than one occasion, to get your HbA1C score down below 7 percent as soon as possible.

With this in mind it reasonable to say that you are in a more serious or critical situation if your HbA1C score is above 7 percent, since you are more likely to develop complications and in a less critical state if your HbA1C score is less than 7 percent, since you would be far less likely to develop complications. Because you are in a more critical state with an HbA1C above 7 percent, it is recommended that you check your blood glucose levels more frequently until such time as you get your score down below 7 percent.

(Table 1 repeated from page 23 for convenience)

Table 1 - Correlation between HbA1C level and mean plasma glucose levels on multiple testing over 2-3 months

Hemoglobin A1C (HbA1C)	Average Blood Glucose (Mg/dl)
13.0%	380
12.0%	345
11.0%	310
10.0%	275
9.0%	240
8.0%	205
7.0%	170
6.0%	135
5.0%	100

When the Hemoglobin A1C is above 7 Percent

Simply put, when your blood glucose levels are running high, you need to test more often. The idea being that by testing more often you will, hopefully, be able to figure out why the blood glucose levels are running high and then make some treatment changes that will bring the blood glucose levels down.

Checking the blood glucose level four times a day, say before each meal and at bedtime would be a good start. For those who would prefer checking their blood glucose levels after meals instead of before, that is also fine. Whether you choose to check your blood glucose levels before or after meals would depend on what you are trying to find out. As an example, if you think your blood glucose may be going too high because of what you ate for breakfast, you need to check it just before you eat and two hours after the start of the meal. If you think your blood glucose level is too high in the late afternoon because of something you ate at lunch, then you need to check it two hours after lunch and just before dinner. If you wake up high in the morning, you need to make sure you check it just before going to bed to see if that had an influence on the morning blood glucose. If you think the blood glucose levels are high because diabetes medications need to be adjusted then testing just before meals is a good time. Again, what you are trying to find out will dictate when you test your blood glucose. There are other scenarios besides the examples here that would require different testing times.

Remember that blood glucose goals before meals should be between 90-130mg/dl., and peak blood glucose levels after meals less than 180mg/dl. Peak blood glucose levels after meals are likely to occur one hour after the start of the meal. Blood glucose readings taken after meals are referred to as post-prandial, whereas blood glucose readings taken before meals are referred to as pre-meal.

For some people it may not make much difference whether they test their blood glucose level before or after they eat. This would likely be the case if the person's blood glucose level was well controlled.

Patients who take insulin injections who have been told by their doctor to adjust the dosage of insulin based on pre-meal blood glucose levels obviously need to go ahead and check their blood glucose levels before the meal. As mentioned previously, if you are curious how high the blood glucose level goes after a meal, then it's a good idea to check the blood glucose level after the meal.

Be careful here though. If you find that the two-hour post-prandial blood glucose levels are too high you may be quick to blame what you ate at the meal as the cause of the post-prandial elevation. But the only way you can accurately determine if what you ate at the meal is the cause of the elevated blood glucose is to know what the blood glucose levels were before the meal. This means checking the blood glucose levels before the meal and again two hours after the start of the meal. If you find the blood glucose level was already high before the meal then the meal may have had little to do with the elevated post-prandial reading. As an example, if the pre meal blood glucose level was 195mg/dl. and the two hour post-prandial blood glucose level was 215mg/dl., then the meal was not responsible for the elevated post-prandial reading. In this case the pre meal blood glucose level was so high that even a light meal, low in carbohydrates, was enough to cause the elevated post-prandial reading.

The best situation for most people would be to vary the schedule. Sometimes check blood glucose levels before meals to see what the levels are, and sometimes check it two hours after meals. In all cases, however, remember to write down in the logbook when the blood glucose reading was taken and the relationship to the nearest meal. As an example, 195mg/dl., 2 1/4 hours post-prandial or 74mg/dl. pre-meal.

It is always wise not to go long periods of time during the day without testing, particularly if the blood glucose levels have been high recently as evidenced either by frequent monitoring or a recent HbA1C.

Consider the following:

Let's say you took three of your closest friends, Nelson, Chloie and Truman, and gave each of them a 300 page book to read. You tell Nelson to read only the first 20 pages of the book. You tell Chloie to read only the middle 20 pages and Truman to read only the last 20 pages. Now you ask them to write a book report. Can they do it? Well they could do it but it wouldn't be very accurate. There would be a lot of guesswork going on because there would be 280 pages that each of them did not read. All three of your friends would be basing their book report only on the 20 pages they had read of a 300-page book. Not only that, each report would be different since each of your friends had read a different 20 pages.

What does this have to do with diabetes and how often to check your blood glucose levels?

Checking blood glucose levels first thing in the morning will only give you information as to what the blood glucose level is right then. You cannot infer from that reading what the blood glucose levels were an hour before or what they are going to be two hours later. The same is true for any other blood glucose reading taken during the day. It only tells you what the blood glucose level is at that very moment. Trying to get an idea how well you have controlled your blood glucose levels during the day by simply checking before breakfast everyday is like trying to write a decent book report after only reading the first twenty pages of the book.

Do you remember when you were younger and connected the dots? You had what looked like a coloring book but before you could color the pages you had to connect the dots to see what the picture was going to be. Once in a while you could see what the picture was going to be before connecting any of the dots. This sometimes happened when there were a lot of dots and they were close together. The pictures where the dots were few and spread out, were the hardest to figure out, because there simply were not enough dots there for you to even begin to make out a pattern. But as you started connecting the dots with lines, you began to get an idea what the picture was going to be. The more dots you connected the more complete the picture became.

Imagine checking your blood glucose at random and infrequently. That's the same thing as having a few dots scattered about the page with no lines between them. You really have no clue what the picture is going to be, nor would you have a clue what is going on with your blood glucose. As you begin connecting the dots that would be analogous to checking your blood glucose more often. Just as the picture would start to appear as you connect more dots you would also be able to get a better understanding of what your blood glucose was doing on a daily basis by testing it more often. The more dots connected the more obvious the picture becomes. The more times you test your blood glucose the clearer it becomes how well or poorly you are controlling your blood glucose levels.

If you have kids you may have once read a book about Carl. (11) Carl is the big, friendly, family dog that is left at home to keep an eye on the baby. On the first page of the book the picture shows the mom dressed and standing by the front door as if she is heading off to work. The picture suggests she says good-bye to Carl who is sitting quietly by the door. The next picture shows her walking down the street. The following pages show Carl going upstairs, getting the baby out of the crib and taking the baby downstairs to the kitchen where they both indulge in a large snack after making a big mess of the kitchen.

Then the two go into the living room, turn on some music and start dancing. Then it's upstairs to mom's room to play dress up.

In the next picture you see is a picture of the clock on the wall indicating that it is a few minutes till 5pm. Carl then takes the baby upstairs bathes the baby, dresses the baby, puts her back in the crib, races downstairs, cleans up all of the messes they made and by two minutes till 5 he goes to the window to look outside for any sign of the mom.

As Carl undoubtedly expected she is walking down the sidewalk approaching the house. In the final picture of the book Carl is standing just inside the door with the mom patting him on the head and saying, "Good dog, Carl." The lady is of the impression that while she was away from the house nothing of any significance occurred. She has no idea what the baby and Carl did while she was gone. And why should she, when she left Carl was standing at the door and when she returned Carl was standing at the door? Things were good when she left and things were good when she returned. Little does she know that just because Carl was waiting for her in the same spot she left him in and just because the house was in the same shape she left it in, that actually quite a bit had gone on that day.

Believe it or not every time I read this story it makes me think of blood glucose monitoring. There have been and still are many people who believe that because their blood glucose levels were good first thing in the morning, maybe around 110mg/dl. and good before dinner, maybe around 115mg/dl., that their blood glucose levels were good all day. Just because Carl was sitting in the same spot when the lady left the house in the morning and when she returned, did that mean that nothing happened all day? Similarly, when you don't check your blood glucose levels during the middle of the day, you really don't have any idea what your blood glucose levels are at that time of day. Knowledge of what the values are at breakfast and dinner provides no information about lunchtime or early afternoon blood glucose levels.

I wrote earlier that before I recommend how often someone should test his or her blood glucose I ask them what their HbA1C score is and make my recommendation based largely on that information. That is definitely true; however, there are several other factors to consider as well. If a person is very elderly or is terminally ill, frequent testing is probably not necessary. Each case should be looked at individually, but in such a case the patient may not be expected to survive long enough for the micro vascular complications associated with diabetes to become too troublesome. Why put the patient through the added burden of frequent blood glucose monitoring?

When a person has no health insurance and has to pay out of pocket for test strips it is often not feasible to test as often. The law mandates that insurance companies pay for testing supplies, and in these cases you are only responsible for the co-payment. In situations when it becomes a real financial burden to test frequently, I recommend only checking four times a day for several days just prior to checkups with your doctor. That way the doctor can review the test results and get some idea what the blood glucose levels have been ranging throughout the day. The assumption here is that the blood glucose values measured over the three to four days prior to seeing the doctor are representative of the blood glucose values over the past several weeks or since the last time any treatment changes were made.

In the meantime testing only once or twice a day may be acceptable. Following this strategy is not the best situation but is acceptable in light of having financial difficulties getting testing supplies for whatever the reason.

When the Hemoglobin A1C is Less Than 7 Percent

When the HbA1C score is less than 7 percent, the risk of developing micro vascular complications decreases. Micro vascular complications are still possible, but the risk is reduced. The lower the score, or the closer you can get to a normal score, the better, as long as you don't find yourself having hypoglycemic episodes, episodes when the level of sugar in the blood drops too low. It may not be necessary to check blood glucose levels more than twice a day when the score is that low. Think about it. With a score of 7 percent or below, we can assume that in most cases the treatment regimen is working, even though it might need a little fine-tuning from time to time to get the score even lower. It is unlikely that you would have many, if any, really "out of control" blood glucose readings with a score of 7 percent or less. As a general rule, unless you are experimenting with new medications or a new treatment regimen, the lower your HbA1C, the less frequently you need to test your blood glucose. Keep in mind that as with many things, there are exceptions to the rule.

For example, if you are going to go do some exercise, it is a good idea to check your blood glucose levels before you begin and when you finish. This is a precautionary measure to help ensure that your blood glucose levels do not drop too low either during or after exercise. This is for safety reasons as well as motivation. I will discuss this in more detail later when I talk about exercise.

Any time you feel peculiar in any way that you cannot explain, or if you are just feeling crummy, you should check your blood glucose. Feeling peculiar may include, but is not limited to, feeling weak, faint, dizzy, light headed, anxious, or nauseated.

Blood glucose levels are also likely to be less stable when you are sick. Glucose levels can sometimes become quite elevated due to the way your body reacts to infections. On the other hand, blood glucose levels can also drop very low, particularly if it is difficult keeping food down. The only way to really know is by checking them more frequently. Because of this someone who usually checks their blood glucose levels two times per day may check their blood glucose level 6-8 times a day when sick. I will discuss this again in more detail later.

Chapter 4
Treating Type 2 Diabetes

When I am teaching a class, before discussing how to best treat type 2 diabetes, I first review with the patients how they most likely developed diabetes and what exactly is wrong with them. I want to make sure they are clear on that before I move on.

I like to start by asking the class, "What is wrong with you? What is not working right inside your body that causes your blood glucose level to go too high? What caused you to develop diabetes?"

"My pancreas quit making insulin, and now I have too much sugar in my blood," is the usual response. It is common for patients to inter mix the term sugar and glucose, which is perfectly acceptable.

Then I ask, "Why did your pancreas stop making insulin?"

"Because I ate too much sugar," they say.

I tell them that if eating too many sweets caused them to gain weight, then, yes it probably did contribute to the development of their diabetes but was probably not the only cause. That was still not the answer I was waiting to hear. Again I ask, "Why did your pancreas, specifically your beta cells, stop producing insulin?" This time I get the answer I was looking for.

"Because the beta cells wore themselves out making all that extra insulin that was needed to get the doors to the cells open."

"What made the doors to the muscle, fat and liver cells so hard to open, I ask?"

"The rusty hinges on the doors," they respond. "It was as if the hinges on the doors to these cells became progressively more rusty over the years, making them increasingly more difficult to open."

"So in the cascade of events that eventually leads to diabetes, where would you say it all starts?" I ask.

"It all starts with the hinges on the doors to the muscle, fat and liver cells getting rusty," they usually say.

"That's right, good job," I tell them. To be clear here, remember that when I refer to the hinges on the doors to the cells becoming rusty, that is really just an analogy meaning that the insulin made in the beta cells of the pancreas has a hard time getting the glucose out of the blood and into the various muscle, fat and liver cells. These cells become progressively more resistant to the effects of insulin over time (insulin resistance) and the insulin sensitivity decreases, leading to steadily increasing amounts of insulin being produced by the beta cells until many beta cells become exhausted and dysfunctional.

Feeling confident that they now have a grasp of what is actually wrong with them, I am now ready to move on to discuss how they can best treat their diabetes. I suggest that if you are still a little confused about this that you go back and reread the section on "how you developed diabetes" as well as the review in the last paragraph. The treatment of diabetes will make a lot more sense if you understand this well.

Optimal Treatment for Type 2 Diabetes

Let's see if you can figure this one out. First, go back and look at what makes the hinges on the doors to the muscle, fat and liver cells rusty. In other words what causes insulin resistance. Do you remember? There are two main causes, a lack of physical activity and being overweight. Just as these are the usual causes for rusty hinges (insulin resistance) getting more exercise and losing some body fat can be, and usually is the best treatment. It is not a cure for diabetes because there is no cure, but diabetes can be controlled to the point of having normal or nearly normal blood glucose levels. Starting to exercise or exercising more if already doing some exercise, plus shedding some fat, can have a profound effect on blood glucose control.

I can think of many occasions when a motivated patient returned to our office 3 months after completing our classes for a follow-up HbA1C to discover that it had dropped from a dangerously high 11 or 12 percent to a 6 or 7 percent. When we ask these patients what they have done to accomplish this big improvement, they usually respond with comments like, "I started walking everyday and cut back on my carbohydrates just like you told me in class. I've lost 25 pounds."

In the case of a patient reducing their HbA1C score from 11 percent to 6 percent, they have gone from having really poorly controlled diabetes to well controlled diabetes in just three months simply by exercising daily, reducing their carbohydrates and losing some weight.

When a patient makes positive changes in his or her eating and exercise habits, these changes are referred to as lifestyle interventions. A little later on I will discuss some research studies that will look at the impact these lifestyle interventions have on preventing diabetes as well as insulin resistance and insulin sensitivity.

Performing regular exercise has the same effect as if you were to take sand paper and sand some of the rust off the rusty hinges, and then spray the hinges with WD-40. With less rust on the hinges, the doors to the cells open a lot easier. As a result the beta cells slow their production of insulin and do not have to continue working so hard. The beta cells like that. Additionally, and equally important, the amount of insulin the remaining beta cells are capable of producing, may be enough to control blood glucose levels with less medicine required and, in some cases, with no medication. This may be true, even if only a fraction of the original number of beta cells are still functioning, and this is particularly true if the patient is also eating wisely.Table 4 - Theoretical amount of insulin needed when insulin resistant and not exercising versus quantity of insulin needed when becoming less insulin resistant due to exercising regularly.

Theoretical amount of insulin needed when insulin resistant and not exercising versus quantity of insulin needed when becoming less insulin resistant due to exercising regularly.

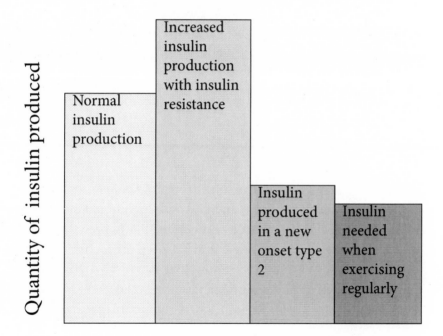

I believe that performing regular aerobic exercise is, without a doubt, the absolute best, most important thing most people can do to prevent diabetes or to improve his or her diabetes if they already have it.

You see, the two best things you can do to prevent developing type 2 diabetes, getting plenty of exercise and losing some excess body fat, if you have it, turn out to be the two best things you can do to treat it once you have it.

I believe so strongly in exercise because of the great results I have personally seen with patients in my office. Even when patients did little else to care for their diabetes besides exercise I could still see big improvements.

I have seen many cases when regular exercise has not resulted in weight loss for my exercising patients but did result in significant improvements in blood glucose control as evidenced by their HbA1C scores. As an example, several years ago, I was asked to come up with some data for an upcoming hospital inspection. Approximately 60 of my patients were surveyed. Twenty-five percent of those surveyed indicated that they had either reduced or eliminated their diabetes medication since starting to exercise. (12)

Improvements in other measurable parameters such as blood pressure, total cholesterol, LDL cholesterol, HDL cholesterol and triglycerides are frequently seen and can be at least partly if not wholly attributed to exercise.

Exercise plays a significant role in lowering blood pressure. About two-thirds of the people with diabetes have high blood pressure, also known as hypertension. Just how much the blood pressure can drop by exercising regularly is unclear and has been the focus of numerous research studies. Scientific studies that have tried to determine this have shown varied results, ranging from both the systolic and diastolic pressure dropping as much as 10mm of Hg to as little as 3.8 and 2.6 mm of Hg, respectively. (13,14) One study found that when exercise was combined with weight loss in men and women with mild hypertension, systolic and diastolic pressure dropped 7.4 and 5.6 mm of Hg., respectively. (15)

It is possible and probably very likely that the magnitude of the drop in systolic and diastolic blood pressure is dependent on several factors. The cause and severity of the hypertension are likely to have something to do with how much the blood pressure drops with exercise, as well as the frequency, duration and intensity of the exercise. When resting blood pressures and blood pressure responses to sub maximal exercise improve as a result of exercise, this is a reflection of improvements in the cardiovascular, muscular and nervous systems.

Similarly, when exercise results in reductions in the various cholesterol levels and triglycerides in the blood, it is due to improvements in mechanisms designed specifically to clear these fats from the blood. The performance of regular exercise appears to enhance the fat clearing mechanisms that help maintain normal or below normal levels of cholesterol and triglycerides in the blood.

Blood Lipids

Exercise has also been shown to have a very favorable effect on blood lipid concentrations.

Although not all studies are in complete agreement, it is generally felt that exercise will reduce levels of total cholesterol, low density cholesterol (LDL's) and triglycerides in the blood while simultaneously raising levels of the beneficial high density cholesterol (HDL's) in the blood. (16) This belief is due in part to the observation that endurance trained athletes have lower total LDL and triglyceride levels in the blood than their more sedentary counterparts. Perhaps the most supportive evidence exists when looking at exercise's ability to reduce blood levels of LDL cholesterol, particularly when combined with weight loss, and triglycerides while at the same time raising levels of HDL cholesterol in the blood. (17,18)

Endurance exercise has been shown to be very effective at lowering triglyceride levels in the blood. (19) The better the control of the triglycerides, the higher the HDL's are likely to be as triglycerides are antagonistic towards HDL's.

With the exception of the HDL cholesterol, which you want to be high, increased levels of any one of these lipids is likely to increase the risk of heart disease and stroke; however, over the years the focus on which of these lipids is most predictive of heart disease and stroke keeps changing.

About 35 years ago, when I first started developing an interest in cholesterol levels, etc., largely due to my dad starting to have a little trouble with his heart, it was total cholesterol levels that physicians were really concerned with when it came to preventing heart disease. Doctors seemed to put a lot of focus on wanting you to get your total cholesterol down. As it turns out a slight reduction in total cholesterol of 1 percent, for example, has been shown to reduce the occurrence of coronary artery disease by 2.5 percent. (20)

Then sometime later the focus shifted to getting the HDL levels up, particularly if the total cholesterol level was too high. The thinking seemed to be that elevated total cholesterol might not be as dangerous if the HDL levels were higher. Doctors started paying attention to the ratio of total cholesterol to HDL cholesterol in the blood.

Then the focus appeared to change once again, now to looking at LDL cholesterol levels and the sub fractions that make up the LDL cholesterol. You see all LDL cholesterol is not the same. There are the small dense LDL particles that are more harmful and the larger "fluffy" LDL particles that are less harmful. The combination of these two sub fractions make up the total LDL cholesterol considered to be "the really bad cholesterol" responsible for clogging up the small arteries that feed the heart. Medications known as "statin" drugs that targeted LDL levels in the blood started being prescribed to patients and for the most part have been successful.

Although exercise can lower levels of this dangerous lipid, it has been suggested that weight loss occurring with exercise will have a more dramatic effect. The goal became to get LDL levels as low as possible to prevent heart disease. This still remains a major goal for many physicians; however, recently there seems to be renewed interest in the importance of raising HDL levels due to their protective effects on the heart. It is fair to say that all of the lipid components mentioned above, plus triglycerides, have a significant impact on the development of heart disease. It is equally important to mention that all can be improved with exercise. (16,17,18,19)

The effects of exercise on raising HDL cholesterol and lowering triglyceride levels in the blood are well documented and of particular interest to patients with diabetes. (16,19)

This is because many patients with type 2 diabetes have lower levels of HDL's in the blood as a result of having high triglyceride levels. You see elevated triglyceride levels lower HDL levels in the blood.

HDL cholesterol is what is commonly referred to as the "good cholesterol." Higher levels of HDL's are thought to have a "protective effect" on the heart and are therefore very desirable. People with higher levels of HDL cholesterol in their blood have a lower risk of developing heart disease or suffering a stroke.

Studies have shown that for every 1 percent increase in HDL levels the risk of heart disease may decrease by as much as 3 percent. (21) Patients with type 2 diabetes frequently have HDL levels that are lower than normal and need to be raised, particularly in light of their increased risk of heart disease.

With the exception of taking the B vitamin, nicotinic acid, shown to be about the only non-exercise means for elevating levels of HDL, besides not smoking if you smoke, exercise is the best bet for increasing this beneficial cholesterol. (22,23) There is evidence to show that at least in women, the more fit they become, the higher their level of HDL cholesterol. (24,25)

Some studies have shown, however, that the lipid lowering and HDL raising benefits of aerobic exercise are not the same for everybody. Some people get better results than others when they initiate an aerobic exercise program. As an example, one study has shown that men with abdominal obesity who have low HDL's and high triglycerides seem to benefit most from regular endurance exercise. This is in contrast to participants in the study with low triglycerides and low HDL's who had a non-significant rise in HDL level with exercise. (26)

Another study, one that reviewed 25 other studies concerning the effects of exercise on HDL levels, showed that the results of such studies often vary due to the duration of the exercise. (27) Exercise frequency and intensity seem to have no significant influence on HDL levels, at least in the 25 studies reviewed. In studies where the weekly energy expenditure was greater than 900 kcal/week or the total exercise time was greater than 120 minutes per week, HDL changes were significant. It also showed that exercise was most beneficial for those with total cholesterol levels over 220mg/dl. and people with a body mass index, (BMI) less than 28.

As for the triglycerides, exercise can significantly reduce their levels in the blood by decreasing insulin resistance, making it easier for the doors to the cells to open so the sugar can get in, and also by decreasing abdominal fat. (28) Excess abdominal fat is associated with a decrease in an enzyme known as lipoprotein lipase (LPL) that limits the breakdown of triglycerides. (29,30)

I also did a search of the literature to see if I could find any research to support my theory that when patients exercise regularly they are more likely to eat better. I am inclined to believe this due to comments I have overheard from patients and also from personal observation, however, with the exception of one study I will mention, I have no scientific proof to support my theory. Perhaps it is because patients feel if they continue to make poor food choices, they will negate all of the benefits derived from the exercise. I suspect that when a patient begins experiencing success with one aspect of their diabetes treatment, such as exercise, and the satisfaction that goes along with it, momentum builds and it may be easier to achieve success in other areas of treatment. Maybe for this reason it is easier to eat better when exercising. For other patients, maybe it is easier for them to make a total commitment to improving their diabetes and they are in the all or nothing mode. As it turned out, my search did find one study showing that when obese women were involved in a supervised aerobic exercise program they demonstrated better dietary compliance. (31)

The author of the study concluded that this additional benefit of aerobic exercise during energy restriction has significant value in the treatment of moderate obesity. With the exception of this study, I found no other evidence to support or refute my theory, however, from what I have seen and heard, I do believe patients eat more healthfully and crave less of the so-called "junk food" when exercising regularly.

Similarly, I have found that the reverse is true. During periods when patients are successfully controlling their caloric intake they are more likely to be successful in their exercise endeavors. This goes along with my "all or nothing" theory.

I stated just recently that I had patients improve their diabetes control simply by exercising, even without losing any weight. How likely is that?

One study involving only women showed that the performance of daily exercise, even without reducing the caloric intake, was associated with substantial reductions in total fat, abdominal fat, visceral fat and insulin resistance. (32) Another study involving 18 sedentary adults, 12 women and 6 men, concluded that even modest amounts of exercise, without weight loss, positively affect glucose and fat metabolism. (33)

I previously discussed, and it is thought by many others, that the reason exercise is critical is that it helps in weight loss and that it is the weight loss that decreases insulin resistance and/or improves diabetes control. This would seem to imply that exercise is only helpful in decreasing insulin resistance because of its contribution to weight loss. As demonstrated by the two studies just cited, however, insulin resistance can be improved with the initiation of exercise and is independent of weight loss.

As I prepared to write this book, it was easy to find research studies that encouraged including exercise as part of the diabetes treatment plan. Most everyone realizes that exercise has value. The problem is that most people do not realize just how much value it has, particularly for people with type 2 diabetes.

I have yet to hear anyone, besides myself that is, come right out and say that exercise is the most important and significant treatment there is for type 2 diabetes! Even the doctors and researchers who promote exercise the most seem to stop short of saying that exercise is the most important treatment for type 2 diabetes. Most articles or summaries of research studies only go so far as to say that exercise should be included as part of an overall treatment plan for controlling diabetes. This, of course is even in light of the considerable evidence supporting the role of exercise in the prevention of insulin resistance and the treatment of type 2 diabetes. (34,35)

I have only recently come across studies that support what I have been telling patients in my classes for years, just how important exercise is. Dr. Ross, in his article, "Does exercise without weight loss improve insulin sensitivity? (36) He states, "There is a growing body of literature indicating that exercise with or without weight loss improves insulin sensitivity." The article goes on to say that since weight loss is known to reverse the insulin resistance that is associated with obesity, (37) and since the performance of regular exercise reduces insulin resistance as well, that the effects of exercise could be magnified if associated with a simultaneous weight/fat loss. (38)

"Combined with the fact that modest exercise reduces the morbidity and mortality associated with cardiovascular disease and diabetes, (39) it is difficult to imagine a more effective therapeutic strategy for reducing insulin resistance and, more importantly, improving overall health and well being." Ekelund, et al. found in his study, (40) that even when increased levels of physical activity produce no changes in aerobic fitness or body fatness, the increased levels of activity may protect against metabolic disease. Ekelund goes on to state, "Therefore, the combination of increasing levels of physical activity and avoidance of gain in fat mass is likely to be the most successful approach for preventing cardiovascular and metabolic disease."

I can tell you now, that after reading through the research as I did, I am as convinced as ever that starting to exercise, or exercising more if already exercising, is the way to go to prevent type 2 diabetes or to treat it if it has already been diagnosed.

Exercise 51, Diet 49

I have told patients that if I had 100 points to divide up between exercise and nutrition (or diet) and I had to give each a number relative to the other indicating their importance when it comes to diabetes control, that I would give exercise 51 points and better nutrition 49. This of course would indicate that I felt exercise played a slightly more important role in diabetes control than nutrition, which of course I do.

My intent in dividing the numbers up this way is not to downplay the significance of better nutrition or shake up the dietitians; I think everyone realizes that nutrition plays a very important role, but to bring to the patients' attention the extreme importance of performing regular exercise. It quite often takes a lot of effort, not just by me but also by the rest of the education staff, to sell the patient on the importance of performing regular exercise. This could be because patients are so often resistant to exercise that they don't want to believe that exercise is so important.

It's as if the patient is saying, "Don't tell me that performing exercise is going to be really good for my diabetes because I really hate to exercise, and I really don't want to hear that." Perhaps they don't like to sweat; maybe they think exercise is too boring, or maybe they have had some unpleasant experiences related to exercise in the past. Remember when exercise was supposed to hurt to be beneficial, as in the expression "no pain, no gain?" That didn't do a lot to get people up and moving. Who is going to want to exercise if it is going to be uncomfortable or hurt every time they do it? Not me. Fortunately, we now know that feeling pain or any significant discomfort during exercise is unnecessary and something to try and avoid. Making patients aware that exercise should not be uncomfortable or produce pain has done a lot to reduce their resistance to exercise.

Need More Doctors to Help

The job of convincing patients with type 2 diabetes just how important it is to exercise could be made a little easier with help from the patients' doctors. As an example, how many times have you heard a doctor say the following, " I think we will try treating this with diet and exercise, initially, and see what happens?" or, " Before we put you on medication, let's try diet and exercise first and see how you do." Both of these are very common statements that physicians or healthcare practitioners treating diabetes are likely to make. Do you notice any similarity between these statements?

In the nearly sixteen years that I have been teaching patients about diabetes I can count on one hand, or more accurately a couple of fingers, the number of times I have heard of a patient being told to try "exercise and diet". The recommendation healthcare people usually make is "diet and exercise". This may not sound like a big deal but it certainly can be.

When a patient is first informed of his or her diagnosis with diabetes, one of the more frequent thoughts that go through the patient's mind is, "That means I can't eat sugar anymore". So I doubt that it is any real surprise to the patient when told by the doctor to try "diet and exercise," as the patient would probably expect the doctor to say something about restricting the sugar intake under the circumstances. Although there is absolutely nothing wrong with saying "diet and exercise", my concern is that when a patient is told to try "diet and exercise," what a lot of patients hear is "DIET and exercise." I think many patients only hear or focus on the diet and not the exercise.

When later questioned by a spouse or family member as to what the doctor recommended as far as treatment for the diabetes, the response is often like this, "The doctor said I have to back off on the amount of sugar I eat, which means less pasta, rolls, rice, fruit and desserts, all the good stuff. I am also supposed to sign up for a diabetes class where I will learn what I can eat that won't cause my blood sugar level to go too high, plus everything else I need to know to take care of diabetes." The patient may not even mention that exercise was discussed.

This may happen for a number of reasons. Maybe the tone of voice the doctor used led the patient to believe that it wasn't as important as the diet. It could be because diet was mentioned before exercise. It could be because the doctor elaborated more on the diet aspect of the recommendation and maybe not at all on the exercise aspect. Maybe the doctor didn't even recommend it because the doctor is unaware of how important it is. Maybe it didn't have anything to do with the way the doctor said it but with what the patient wanted to hear or was willing to hear. Regardless of the reason, what the newly diagnosed patient needed to hear and understand was that exercise was extremely important in maintaining control of the diabetes. Unfortunately, that is not the message the patient came home with.

Why can't we say "exercise and diet" instead of "diet and exercise"? Maybe that would work better at getting the point across. Maybe that would work better at getting patients to exercise. If doctors and healthcare providers recommended exercise more strongly, it might not make any difference, which comes first. However, with the way things are now, where the vast majority of patients with diabetes do not realize the significance of exercise, measures must be taken to make it clear.

Doctors could help patients a great deal by taking a moment to inquire as to the patient's past and present exercise habits and then to explain very briefly how important it is to exercise. The doctor doesn't need to go into detail as long as he or she gets the point across to the patient that exercise can be very effective. Ideally the doctor would discuss exercise just enough so that when the patient walks out of the exam room the patient is thinking, "Gee, doing some exercise must be a really big deal the way the doctor talked about it. The doctor makes it sound like it is the best thing I can do for my diabetes. I think I better start exercising tonight!"

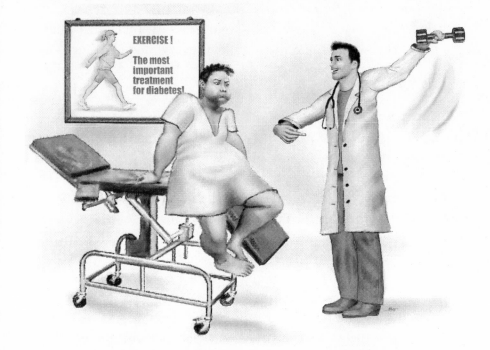

Doctors could be tremendously helpful to their patients by enthusiastically recommending that they exercise.

For a lot of patients in my parents' generation; they are both in their early 80's, whatever the doctor says, goes. Many of these people put their health matters in their doctor's hands and trust the doctor to make the right decision, often times not even asking questions. I believe that with this segment of the population if the doctor would just simply tell the patient what exercise to do, the patient may be very likely to do it just because the doctor said so!

Why Exercise Earns More Points Than Diet

You probably want to know why I gave exercise 51 points while only giving better nutrition 49 when I have already stated how both "lifestyle interventions" are so very important in controlling diabetes. What is it about exercise that makes me believe it is more important than better nutrition and the overall best treatment for type 2 diabetes? In about four out of five cases of type 2 diabetes, insulin resistance (rusty hinges) is the cause. As a result of insulin resistance the beta cells respond by making considerably more insulin than normal until many of them eventually wear out and become dysfunctional. The cause of insulin resistance (rusty hinges) is most always a lack of physical activity, being over fat, or a combination of both.

Studies have shown that initiating an exercise program or increasing present levels of physical activity can improve insulin resistance, and studies have shown that reducing bodyweight or excess body fat will improve insulin resistance as well.

As for losing weight as a means of reducing insulin resistance, does it matter what the weight consists of and does it matter how it is lost? These are two very important questions and the answer to at least one of these questions has a lot to do with the results obtained when the weight comes off.

First of all, does it matter where the weight comes from and what the weight consists of?

It most definitely does matter. People are most often considered overweight if they weigh more than is expected for their height. If the reason for being overweight is because the person is heavily muscled, possibly due to lifting weights or participation in athletics and sports, that is not a problem. Neither insulin resistance nor diabetes results from a person carrying too much muscle. The problem with height and weight tables as well as body mass index calculations (BMI) is that they fail to take into account the amount of muscle the person carries on their frame.

Conversely, if people are overweight because they carry excessive fat on their bodies, then insulin resistance results and gets progressively worse as the fat on the body increases. As an example, probably most, if not all, bodybuilders would be considered overweight because of the greater than normal quantity of muscle they have built on their bodies. Typically, body builders who may be considered overweight according to BMI tables, would have body fat percentages down in the 2-5 percent range. Someone else of the same height and weight as a bodybuilder, but who is mostly sedentary, may also be classified by a table or formula as being overweight. In the case of this person, however, due to lower levels of physical activity and possibly overeating, the person is overweight due to carrying an excess amount of body fat. This person may have a percent body fat of 30 percent or more, in sharp contrast to the 2-5 percent body fat of the bodybuilder. It is, therefore, fair to say that not all of the methodologies used to assess a person's body fatness are accurate.

Secondly, does it make a difference how a person takes the weight off? Can it be done by cutting calories or by getting more exercise?

It doesn't seem to matter, according to Dr. Ed Weiss and colleagues at St. Louis University. (41) In their study, at the end of one year, weight loss was the same whether it was accomplished by cutting calories or by continuing to eat as always but adding exercise. Both the exercise group and the calorie-cutting group saw improvements in insulin resistance and insulin sensitivity. What Dr. Weiss did not look at in this study but would like to know is whether the combination of cutting calories and exercise would provide even better results versus each intervention separately? A later study by Weiss and colleagues in 2006, indicated there was no greater improvement in insulin resistance when exercise alone produced weight loss versus when weight loss occurred from caloric restriction. (42)

If it doesn't matter how the weight is lost, then patients should be able to choose the method that works best for them…right?

Not necessarily, it's not quite that simple. Although calorie cutting alone or with the addition of exercise may both get some much needed weight off, what's to say it will stay off? After all, many long time dieters know that keeping the weight off is the real challenge. They may have lost weight on numerous occasions only to gain it all back plus sometimes more. Bret Goodpaster, PhD., exercise physiologist and assistant professor of medicine at the University of Pittsburgh, believes this is where exercise can be the most helpful, helping to keep the weight off once it is lost. "When weight loss does occur through caloric restriction, in order to maintain the weight loss and the improved insulin sensitivity that goes along with it, utilizing exercise to build muscle may help "train" the body to use dietary fat more efficiently. When it comes to weight loss exercise is more for helping people maintain the loss and prevent regain." (43)

So, if weight loss, regardless of how it occurs, decreases insulin resistance and improves insulin sensitivity; and if Dr. Goodpaster's theory is correct, that exercise is necessary to keep lost weight off, it should be clear why I say exercise is so important, even a little bit more important than better nutrition.

Any factor that contributes to reduced insulin resistance and improved insulin sensitivity, in this case exercise and weight loss or the combination of both, is likely to make life easier for those beta cells still functioning (reduce the workload of the beta cells) and may slow the rate at which remaining beta cells become dysfunctional.

There are five big reasons why I believe exercise is at least as important as good nutrition, if not more so, when it comes to diabetes control.

1. With weight loss comes reduced insulin resistance and improved insulin sensitivity, both very desirable. Regardless of the method used to lose weight, whether it is caloric restriction or

increased physical activity, the performance of regular exercise has been proposed to be necessary to maintain weight loss. In other words whatever weight is lost is likely to return if exercise is not started and maintained. For this reason alone, the performance of regular exercise, for any patient trying to lose weight and keep it off, would seem to be absolutely necessary and at least as important as improved nutrition. But wait there's more.

2. The performance of regular exercise is known to reduce levels of total cholesterol, LDL cholesterol and triglycerides, in the blood while simultaneously raising the levels of HDL's in the blood. Higher levels of HDL's in the blood reduce the risk of heart disease and stroke. While restricting the intake of saturated fats and sugars may also lead to improvements in the lipid profile, (reduced triglycerides and increased HDL's), exercise provides a means to clear excess levels of these fats out of the blood and may be very useful at doing this when dietary compliance is not at its best.

3. Exercise is a safe and effective means to lower blood pressure. Sometimes in cases of mild high blood pressure exercise is all that is necessary to bring blood pressure readings down to normal levels. Sometimes exercise in conjunction with medications is necessary to get blood pressures under good control. Reducing salt, and perhaps caffeine intake, are really the only nutrition interventions known to have a favorable impact on lowering blood pressure.

4. For patients who continually have difficulty reducing the amount of carbohydrates they consume, either at mealtime or in between, leading to significant elevations in blood glucose readings, performing exercise at these times can be an effective means to at least partially compensate for these dietary indiscretions.

5. The performance of regular exercise may increase a patient's motivation to eat better, lose weight, take medications on time, and generally take better care of their diabetes. Never underestimate the importance of exercise when it comes to improving a patient's overall feeling of well being. This may be associated with my theory

that patients with type 2 diabetes eat more healthfully when they are exercising regularly.

That's it, the five big reasons I believe exercise is just a little bit more important than nutrition and the most significant treatment for type 2 diabetes.

On one hand, pointless to make that determination if a patient is already planning a well rounded approach to his or her diabetes care; but on the other hand, vitally important if a patient thought simply cutting down on carbohydrates and generally eating healthier were enough to take care of the diabetes. Trust me it usually is not!

I always like to tell my patients in class, that if the only thing they learn after their ten hours of class is that they need to exercise nearly every day of the week, if not daily, and then they make that behavioral change, the cost of the class and the ten hours they spent in class were well worth it. They have gotten the main message.

Perhaps you have heard the expression, "A man's man" when referring to someone, hopefully a male, or the phrase, "The best of the best", when describing a very elite group of people. With this in mind I suggest the following, "that exercise is the most important of the important treatments" when it comes to treating type 2 diabetes. I say this knowing full well that not all diabetes educators will agree with this; that there are likely doctors and some endocrinologists that may not agree. As for these people, I just have more convincing to do. Some non-believers may be quick to point to a 2006 study that summarized the results of 27 other studies and concluded that performing aerobic exercise, resistance exercise, or a combination of the two, leads to only "trivial" changes in HbA1C scores for training lasting more than 12 weeks. The reduction in HbA1C was only 0.8 ± 0.3 percent. (44) Unfortunately, this may be all some people need to hear to justify their continued sedentary lifestyle.

Now, considering that for each one percent drop in HbA1C the onset of micro vascular complications is reduced by 37 percent, as well as a 14 percent reduction in myocardial infarctions (heart attacks), a 0.8 percent reduction seems pretty worthwhile to me.

Additionally, you want to be careful not to judge the effectiveness of exercise by simply looking at HbA1C scores alone. The HbA1C is just one of many measurable parameters that should improve with regular exercise. It would be a huge mistake to not also look at blood pressure changes, lipids and changes in body composition, all of which are likely to improve with regular exercise.

Nevertheless, there will undoubtedly be skeptics, those who still undervalue the many benefits regular exercise has to offer for the person with diabetes. My hunch is, though, that the skeptics have never put exercise to the test. They have never given it a good try; that is, approached exercise with enthusiasm and really put some effort into getting the patients they care for to try it.

I started to write, "That's alright, one day they will come around," but, really, it is not all right; it is very unfortunate that patients are missing out on this important treatment. I am hopeful that more health professionals will come around, soon, and begin more enthusiastically recommending that patients engage in a program of regular physical activity or exercise. Aside from anecdotal success stories I could tell you about from patients in my office, there are the research studies. As for me, I typically wouldn't make a change in something I did or didn't do simply because of anecdotal success stories; I would want to see some research to support making the change. Many people are like me in this regard. Fortunately, there seems to have been greater interest in exercise in the past ten years and an increase in the number of research studies involving exercise and nutrition. It is gratifying to see so much of the research confirming what I have observed in my patients for years, that exercise can make such a big difference. It's also encouraging to see more studies being conducted looking at "lifestyle interventions," such as exercise and better nutrition, in the prevention and treatment of type 2 diabetes, particularly concerning resistance training. After reading some of the recent research about exercise and what it can do for the treatment of type 2 diabetes, maybe you too will become enthusiastic in believing that exercise is so very important.

With the knowledge that weight loss, whether due to caloric restriction or increased exercise activity, improves insulin resistance and is therefore important in the treatment of type 2 diabetes, do you think these two lifestyle interventions may play a role in preventing insulin resistance, pre diabetes or diabetes? To investigate the theory that lifestyle intervention can play a critically important role in preventing diabetes or positively affecting impaired glucose tolerance, studies were conducted to specifically investigate this issue.

The Da Quing study (34) involved 577 people with impaired glucose tolerance identified by population-based screening in Da Quing, China. Two hundred and eighty four of these people were randomized to undergo a diet change and/or increased physical activity. Insulin resistance (IR) and insulin sensitivity (IS) were assessed. The interactions of IR, IS, obesity and plasma glucose under the influence of the lifestyle intervention were evaluated. After following the participants for 6 years, the results showed that both IR and IS were significantly associated with the development of diabetes. Diet plus exercise interventions resulted in a significantly lower incidence of diabetes. Both insulin resistance and beta cell function were predictors of diabetes in Chinese with impaired glucose tolerance (IGT). Lifestyle intervention reduced the incidence of diabetes and was more effective in those with less IR.

The Finnish Diabetes Prevention Study (DPS) (35) involved 522 middle-aged, overweight individuals with impaired glucose tolerance (IGT) and was one of the first controlled randomized studies to show that type 2 diabetes is preventable with lifestyle intervention. The risk of developing type 2 diabetes was reduced by 58 percent in the intensive lifestyle intervention group that included both improved nutrition and exercise therapy, compared with the control group. Also significant about this study is that one of the main objectives was to test an intervention that was feasible in primary healthcare.

Possibly the most well known study to look at lifestyle interventions is the Diabetes Prevention Program (DPP). (45) This study was designed to determine the effectiveness of either lifestyle intervention or pharmacological therapy in the prevention or delay of type 2 diabetes in people with impaired glucose tolerance (IGT), that are at high risk for diabetes. The results showed that both the lifestyle intervention and pharmacological treatment were successful in reducing new cases of diabetes; however, the lifestyle intervention group decreased the incidence of new cases by 58 percent, whereas the group treated pharmacologically with metformin only experienced a reduction of 31 percent. The reduction of 58 percent seen here with the lifestyle intervention group is, interestingly, the same as observed in the Finnish study. It is important to note that the lifestyle intervention employed in this study involved considerable assistance from health professionals for support, encouragement, counseling, etc., and would not be appropriate for use in the community.

The above-mentioned studies make it clear that lifestyle interventions can prevent or at least delay the onset of type 2 diabetes. What is not clear from the studies, however, is what part of the intervention, improved nutrition, exercise, or both, was responsible.

Lending support to the notion that exercise, independent of diet, has a lot to do with the risk reduction of developing type 2 diabetes, in 2002 a review of studies published between 1990 and 2000 concluded that the reduction in the risk of type 2 diabetes associated with a physically active, compared with a sedentary, lifestyle is 30-50 percent and that physical activity provides a similar risk reduction for coronary heart disease (CHD). (46)

Additionally, the performance of regular physical activity may slow the initiation and progression of type 2 diabetes and its associated cardiovascular complications due to its positive effects on body weight, insulin sensitivity (IS), blood glucose control, blood pressure, lipid profile, fibrinolysis, endothelial function and inflammatory defense systems. (46)

People with impaired glucose tolerance (IGT) are in sort of a gray area, that is, their blood glucose levels are not normal but are also not elevated enough to meet the criteria for having diabetes. Once having IGT, short of making some significant changes in lifestyle, the odds are that these people will eventually progress to having diabetes. Probably one of the best reasons for carrying out the above-mentioned studies is to answer the question asked by so many people diagnosed with IGT, "Can someone diagnosed with IGT ever go back to achieving normal blood glucose levels, or is he or she always going to eventually end up with diabetes?" These studies not only demonstrate that insulin resistance (IR) and insulin sensitivity (IS) can both be improved with exercise, but also prove that people with IGT have the ability to correct the disorder and postpone or prevent ever developing diabetes.

More studies need to be done that will better distinguish the benefits of each lifestyle intervention, independently of the other, and combined. I would postulate that the greatest reduction in diabetes risk occurs when the patient employs both lifestyle interventions; that, of course, being better nutrition and exercise. Second to that, I think starting an exercise program or increasing the amount of exercise would show the next greatest reduction followed by better nutrition.

One of the things I discuss and illustrate for patients in class is the concept I showed previously. That is, I show them how much insulin is produced in a normal situation when a standard amount of sugar is dumped into the blood. I then show them how much insulin is needed when the patient is insulin resistant, which is a good bit more than in the person that is not insulin resistant. Next, I show them the limited quantity of insulin capable of being produced in a new onset type 2, approximately half the normal amount. It is because of this reduction in insulin production that the patient has to compensate by restricting their carbohydrate intake and take diabetes medication. The final column in the graph shows the amount of insulin a patient may need after they have started exercising regularly. I point out to the patients that the third column is pretty much always going to be larger than the fourth column indicating that even when insulin production is limited, when a patient engages in regular exercise, it is conceivable that the amount of insulin required is less than the amount produced.

This is consistent with what I observed and stated earlier that at one point 25 percent of my patients surveyed had either eliminated or reduced the amount of diabetes medication they were taking since starting to exercise. (12)

In summary, the two controllable risk factors that typically lead to type 2 diabetes, weight gain in the form of body fat and lack of exercise, when corrected, can reduce insulin resistance and the likelihood of developing pre diabetes and diabetes. If pre diabetes, IGT, has been diagnosed, it is possible that with immediate lifestyle changes the development of type 2 diabetes could be averted or at least postponed. Once type 2 diabetes has been diagnosed, engaging in more physical activity or exercise and eating more healthfully are frequently the very best things to do.

Chapter 5
Exercise

Have you ever opened a gift or taken a product out of the box it came in and found that when you started to read the instructions the first line said something like, "Congratulations on your recent purchase of this fine piece of merchandise. Proper care and use of this product will provide you with hours of fun and excitement."

For those folks choosing exercise as a major treatment option for the care of their diabetes, I want to say, congratulations on selecting exercise as your treatment of choice. Performing regular exercise as outlined below is likely to provide you with days, weeks and years of much improved blood sugar control.

In the following pages I will tell you pretty much all you should need to know to get you going on your exercise program.

Before I start discussing exercise recommendations for patients who should exercise, I need to point out that some patients with diabetes, unfortunately, should not exercise. These are frequently patients with advanced stages of heart disease and/or other co-morbid conditions. A co-morbid condition is another co-existing serious life threatening medical condition.

The increased work the heart must do during exercise can be too much for a diseased heart. If these patients are to exercise, it would be wise to do it in a cardiac rehabilitation setting under the guidance of professionals trained to work with patients with more advanced heart disease.

Fortunately, the number of patients who should not exercise because it poses too great a risk is very small, and the vast majority of people with diabetes can and should exercise regularly. To find out if exercise is safe for you, it is always a good idea to get checked out by your doctor first. I sincerely mean this. Keep in mind that just having diabetes is a major risk factor for heart disease, and it is estimated that two out of three people with diabetes will die from heart disease or stroke. (1) With this in mind, I mean it when I say that a doctor's approval should be obtained before beginning an exercise program.

The heart health of anyone wanting to start an exercise program needs to be known so the appropriate steps can be taken to better ensure the participant's safety during exercise.

Patients with known heart disease or newly diagnosed heart disease can usually exercise, and it is frequently recommended once the doctor has treated the patient and the patient follows the appropriate guidelines. In the facility where I supervised the exercise program, physician clearance was required before I allowed patients to join the program. Because of the high prevalence of heart disease with type 2 diabetes, if the patient has a cardiologist, it is recommended the patient get clearance from that doctor.

In some cases a doctor will not give clearance until a cardiovascular workup is completed, including a stress test. I leave that up to the doctor to decide whether the patient needs a stress test or not. Healthcare professionals have debated whether a stress test is really necessary prior to the initiation of exercise in various populations. There are good arguments for and against it; however, in the end, every effort should be made to ensure the safety of the patient. For now, the most recent clinical practice recommendations, according to the American Diabetes Association, state that a graded exercise test with electrocardiogram (ECG) monitoring should be seriously considered before undertaking aerobic physical activity with intensity exceeding the demands of everyday living (more intense than brisk walking) in a previously sedentary person with diabetes whose 10-year risk of a coronary event is likely to be greater than or equal to 10 percent. (47) An advantage of having a stress test, if recommended, is that if this is your first one, it can serve as a baseline for all other stress tests to be compared against. It can also be motivational if you find that with each successive stress test you take your performance improves or remains unchanged, as you get older.

A disadvantage of having a stress test is the likelihood of having a false positive test result. A false positive test is when the test shows that there is something wrong when really there is nothing wrong. Aside from getting the patient all worked up, false positive tests often lead to invasive testing, such as a cardiac catheterization, designed to confirm or rule out the suspected problem. The problem with invasive tests is that they cannot be performed without a certain degree of risk to the patient.

For this reason, the U.S. Preventive Services Task Force recently concluded that stress tests should not routinely be recommended for people who are not experiencing any symptoms of heart disease and are generally at low risk of having heart disease. It was felt that the risk of doing a cardiac catheterization was greater than the benefit obtained by detecting previously unidentified ischemia. (48,49)

Exercise Recommendations

Before I get into my thoughts on exercise, what I have observed with patients and what I recommend, I will share with you the official guidelines established by the most recognized professional organizations.

After you read them I believe we will agree that the guidelines are very similar and say pretty much the same thing, that exercise should be done for a minimum of 30 minutes daily if possible, and if not daily almost everyday. Take a look.

The U.S. Surgeon General's Report recommended that most people accumulate greater than or equal to 30 minutes of moderate intensity exercise on most, ideally all, days of the week. (50)

The American College of Sports Medicine and Centers for Disease Control recommend that all adults in the United States accumulate 30 minutes or more of moderate-intensity physical activity on most if not all days of the week. (51)

The Clinical Practice Recommendations of the ADA on Physical Activity state that to improve blood glucose control, assist with weight maintenance, and reduce the risk of cardiovascular disease, at least 150 min per week of moderate-intensity aerobic physical activity (50-70 percent of maximum heart rate) is recommended and/or at least 90 minutes per week of vigorous aerobic exercise (>70 percent of maximum heart rate). The physical activity should be distributed over at least 3 days per/week and with no more than two consecutive days without physical activity. (47)

The American College of Sports Medicine Position Stand on Exercise and Type 2 Diabetes states that people with type 2 diabetes should try to utilize a minimum of 1000 kcal per week through physical activity or exercise. (52)

In the absence of contraindications, people with type 2 diabetes should also be encouraged to include resistance exercise as part of their exercise program. The most common form of resistance exercise is usually considered to be lifting weights, also known as weight training. This type of exercise should be done three times per week, targeting all major muscle groups progressing to three sets of 8-10 repetitions at a weight that cannot be lifted in good form more than 8-10 times. (47) The American College of Sports Medicine now recommends that resistance training be included in fitness programs for adults with type 2 diabetes. (52) Two clinical trials published in 2002 provided strong evidence for the value of resistance training in type 2 diabetes. (53,54) Research has shown that one reason for falls in older adults is a lack of strength.

Maintaining reasonable levels of overall body strength in older adults may help prevent accidents and falls, and ultimately improve the quality of life. Different guidelines are usually recommended depending on the health and goals of the patient.

So, with the exception of the position stand on exercise and type 2 diabetes, the guidelines are all pretty much in agreement.

In regards to the position stand on Exercise and Type 2 Diabetes, after a patient adapts to the initial stresses of starting an exercise program, if the patient is satisfied exercising just enough to meet the minimum caloric expenditure requirement of 1000 kcal per week, I am very doubtful the patient will ever realize anywhere near the full potential of what exercise has to offer. This position stand seems to be the most lenient of all the exercise recommendations, as a caloric expenditure of 1000 kcal per week is on the lower end of the scale. There are many cases when I would recommend to my patients that once they are comfortable with a 1000 caloric expenditure of calories through exercise, they try to work towards a 2000 calorie expenditure of calories.

Although the amount of exercise a person with type 2 diabetes needs to do to maximize its many benefits has yet to be determined, it is reasonable to believe that the benefits will increase as the amount of exercise increases, to a point.

I have been fortunate to be a diabetes educator for approximately 16 years now and had the rewarding experience of witnessing hundreds and hundreds of exercise sessions of patients with diabetes. The observations and suggestions I make concerning exercise in this section are the result of what I have learned through my experiences with these patients and witnessing their many exercise sessions.

Exercise Prescription

Anytime anybody starts becoming more physically active than they were before, they are doing a good thing, a really good thing. Some patients don't want to be bothered with a bunch of exercise guidelines, but they are willing to agree to become more physically active. In these cases I simply offer suggestions as to how he or she can become more physically active. Now, the patient's ideas of how they can become more physically active and my idea of how they can become more physically active are not always the same and, unfortunately, I cannot always get the patients to see it my way. However, as long as the patients are willing to be more physically active than they had been previously, they are better off. Sometimes I have to leave it at that.

Then there are those who want me to tell them what to do, how long to do it, how often to do it and how vigorously. That's where the exercise prescription comes in. An exercise prescription is when I explain to a patient what type of exercise to do, how long to exercise, how often to exercise, and how vigorously to exercise. Professionals refer to this as the type, duration, frequency and intensity of exercise.

Doctors sometimes give a patient some or all of this information, but not often. If a physician does happen to recommend exercise to a patient, it is often without any real guidelines. Exercise is like any other medicine; if taken according to directions and used properly, it works well; if taken incorrectly, it can be very dangerous. Without real guidelines, well meaning, enthusiastic patients may go out and over exert themselves, either by exercising too long or too vigorously. This over exertion could result in some serious long-term consequences.

As an example, if an injury results, such as a sprain, strain, shin splints (pain occurring on the front side of the shin), or stress fracture, the exercise regimen would be temporarily halted while the injury heals. Since many people with diabetes, as well as many that are older, take longer to heal, this injury may keep the patient sidelined for as little as a couple of days to as long as several weeks or even months depending on the severity of the injury.

Another consequence of starting off too vigorously and overdoing it is that if this causes some noticeable muscle discomfort (stiffness, soreness, cramping, etc.) and this person has traditionally been a non-exerciser and is not accustomed to muscle discomfort or soreness, the person may say, "I don't want to do this, this hurts! My legs hurt for three days after I walked." In this case although the person did not experience any significant injury, the negative feelings associated with the three days of muscle soreness may be enough to seriously dampen their desire to exercise, enough so that the person does not pursue it any further. This probably could have been prevented if the person had been given appropriate guidelines for starting a walking or exercise program.

Exercise professionals such as physical therapists and exercise physiologists frequently explain the four components that make up an exercise prescription, making it clear.

Type of Exercise

When embarking on a new exercise program, it is essential that to choose exercises that accomplish the goals you have in mind. If someone wants to train to run a three-mile road race, doing forearm exercises in the gym is of little value. If someone wants to get rid of some body fat that has accumulated around the waist, doing three different types of sit ups will be of little value.

Unfortunately, when left on their own, many people are not able to design a program that is best suited to meet their goals. I overheard a lady at the YMCA say just this morning that she is just getting into "this" (meaning going to the gym) after quitting smoking. She was telling an older couple, that had just complimented her on her hard work, that she was trying to do the exercises she had seen other people do in the gym, because she really didn't know what to do. I think this happens a lot. If you are impressed by someone's physique, you do what he or she is doing and you will up looking like him or her, right? Probably not, there is often a lot more to it than that.

Aerobic or Anaerobic?

Aerobic: The definition of aerobic exercise is "with oxygen" or "requiring oxygen".

Very short bursts of physical activity or exercise do not require oxygen. These are activities generally lasting up to a maximum of a couple of minutes. Now to be clear on this, yes, you must keep breathing during this time, but your body has alternative ways of generating fuel for your muscles to work without oxygen, but only for very short periods of time, like approximately two minutes or less.

For an exercise to be considered aerobic, generally, the exercise needs to involve large muscle groups used in a rhythmic fashion for more than several minutes at a time. It is also recommended that the heart rate be raised somewhat above resting levels during the exercise, however, not to excessively high levels. In some cases patients may not be able to exercise for more than several minutes at a time when first getting started. That's perfectly all right. In these situations the patients do what they can do without causing any significant discomfort. As time goes on when their body adapts to the physical stresses of exercise, they become stronger and are gradually able to do more.

Walking, cycling and swimming are excellent choices of aerobic exercise. I listed these first because they seem to be the most popular and easiest to do, particularly as we get older. Whether you choose to walk outdoors or on a treadmill is entirely up to you and makes little difference as far as the benefit. Similarly, cycling can be performed on a stationary bike or outdoors on the road. As you can imagine, it is safer doing it on a stationary bike because there is no traffic; however, unless you are peddling that stationary bike in front of a television, or you are listening to music, or you have someone to talk to while you ride, stationary cycling can be a little, well, less than exciting. Swimming is great as it uses most all of your major muscle groups. There are also numerous other examples of aerobic exercise including racquetball, dancing, tennis, soccer, basketball, skating, jogging, etc.

Anaerobic (resistance training): Anaerobic exercise can be defined as "without oxygen". These would be activities requiring quick bursts of energy which can be accomplished in as little as 2-3 seconds or might last as long as 90-120 seconds. Examples include resistance training (weight lifting and weight machines), push-ups, sit-ups, pull-ups, or even running to the house from the car to get out of the rain!

Until fairly recently, aerobic exercise was the preferred type of exercise for patients with type 2 diabetes. Anaerobic exercise, such as weight lifting, often referred to as resistance training, was not usually encouraged and actually sometimes discouraged as it was not thought to be as beneficial as aerobic exercise and could actually be considered harmful for patients with high blood pressure and eye disease (retinopathy). Although performing any exercise, be it aerobic or resistance training, can be dangerous and is not recommended when a patient's blood pressure is not under good control, resistance training has recently been shown to be very effective in improving many of the parameters adversely affected by diabetes. (9,10,14)

In fact, in a study of 62 Latino adults, (40 men and 22 women) resistance training was not only shown to lower systolic blood pressures (The systolic blood pressure is the pressure at which the blood is ejected from the left ventricle of the heart and into the aorta) but to also reduce their diabetes medication by 72 percent as compared to the control group that did no resistance training and whose diabetes medications increased by 42 percent. (54)

In a study of older men in their sixties with type 2 diabetes, performing resistance training as little as two times per week was enough to show a decrease in abdominal fat and improve insulin sensitivity. (55)

One study was able to sum up the majority of benefits derived from resistance training nicely by stating in the conclusion that resistance training significantly improved blood glucose control, increased fat free mass, reduced the need for diabetes medications, reduced abdominal fat and systolic blood pressure, and increased muscle strength and spontaneous physical activity. (54) As for the concern that resistance training may aggravate diabetes related eye disease (retinopathy), causing the rupture of more small vessels in the retina, it is not likely to happen if the patient avoids excessive straining, has well controlled blood pressures, and has no active bleeding.

Aerobic and Anaerobic: Fueled in part by the previously mentioned studies supporting the inclusion of resistance training as part of a diabetes management plan, resistance exercise should now be recommended routinely in addition to aerobic exercise in the exercise prescription. An exception to this, of course, would be a preexisting medical condition when resistance training would be a known contraindication. The resistance exercise should include all major muscle groups, be performed three times per week, and eventually progressing to three sets of 8-10 repetitions at a weight that cannot be lifted more than 8-10 times. (47)

Excessive straining and breath holding should always be avoided since both practices could be dangerous. As far as how much rest to take between sets, generally speaking, one to one and a half minutes between sets should be sufficient for most people. If this does not seem to be enough, then it is possible the amount of weight being lifted is too much and should be reduced. When first getting started it would be wise to only perform one set of each exercise for maybe the first two weeks, two sets of each exercise for maybe the third and fourth week and progress to three sets when two sets is not producing any significant soreness.

The idea here is to progress slowly. Extra care should always be taken if you are way out of shape and very poorly conditioned. Always let your doctor know if you plan on doing anything more strenuous than routine daily activities. That way the doctor can make you aware of any specific precautions you should take, etc.

I could go on and on here, but the fact is, the combination of aerobic exercise and anaerobic exercise (resistance training) is the way to go for most people trying to realize the greatest benefits exercise has to offer.

Choosing an Aerobic Exercise: When many people think of aerobic exercise, they think of walking, swimming or riding a bike.

That's good since all are excellent choices. Which is the best though? That's a good question, and one that I get asked a lot. What do you think? Which one is best if you are trying to lose weight? Walking, maybe, because it is weight bearing (meaning you have to support your weight while doing it) and will therefore cause you to burn the greatest amount of calories in the shortest period of time. How about if you have knee problems and walking hurts your knee? Swimming, maybe, because it is non-weight bearing (you are not supporting your weight) and it may not bother your knee. What about if you have neuropathy (damage to the nerves in the feet and lower body), again, swimming may be the best choice as it is non-weight bearing. With neuropathy, weight bearing exercise is usually discouraged due to the risk of doing damage to the feet. .

These are all good ideas that have worked for many people. So why do I keep saying, "maybe"? Because, although all are good choices, given the conditions, but what if the patient who would benefit from walking doesn't like to walk? Then walking is not a good choice for that person. If cycling is recommended, but you really find cycling to be boring, then don't do it, choose something else. Selecting an aerobic exercise that you have tried in the past but did not like is probably not a great plan. After much discussion in class, I ultimately tell the class that the best exercise is the one they are most likely to do, the one that they like the most.

What you are looking for is aerobic exercise that you can do and one that you like, maybe not as much as a good book or having your back rubbed, but an aerobic activity that doesn't cause you to snarl or curse or sigh at its very mention.

One time a patient asked me which exercise burned the most calories per minute, the idea being that since her main objective was to lose weight she wanted to do the exercise that burned the most calories. I told her that of the equipment she had available to her the stair climber was her best bet.

The patient slapped her hand against my desk with disgust and replied, "Oh geez, I hate that one!"

Then, after a big sigh she told me, "Okay, I guess I will do that one then. I was hoping you were going to say walking because I love to walk."

I told her to walk then and to forget the stair climber. Even though the patient may burn more calories per minute using a stair climber versus a treadmill, if she doesn't like stair climbing, she has no business doing it. That would not be a good idea. She might will herself to stair climb, initially, but in a very short period of time, as her motivation waned, her stair climbing days would be over. I told her that even if walking burned fewer calories per minute than stair climbing she would be far better off walking because she liked to walk and would be more likely to do it on a regular basis.

One of my patients tells me outright that he does not like to exercise and that he looks forward to the weekends when he doesn't have to come to my office and do it. That is because we are closed on weekends. The same gentleman rarely misses a workout and usually comes in at least four days per week. This patient has been coming in for more than three years now. If in fact this patient hates to exercise as much as he says he does, this would be a very rare situation. It would be extremely rare for a patient to come in and exercise with regularity for three years if the patient really disliked exercise that much. My guess is the patient didn't mind exercising as much as he said he did. In fact I think he actually liked coming in and socializing with the other patients while he exercised.

I believe that with few exceptions, for an exercise program to continue long term, allowing the patient to derive all of the many benefits of exercise, there must be something pleasurable or rewarding associated with actually doing the exercise. As an example, I have seen adults get really enthusiastic about cycling. They try it a few times and find that they really like the feeling they get when going 40 miles per hour down a steep hill. I have seen others get hooked on cycling because they like all the high tech gadgetry and components on the bikes and the flashy clothing they get to wear.

Think about it, under what other circumstances is it acceptable for a grown man to walk into a convenience store to get a Powerbar wearing multicolored, skin tight spandex shorts and a shirt (the correct term is jersey) with a super hero looking bicycle helmet on his head except because he is a cyclist? As an aside, and this has absolutely nothing to do with diabetes and is not meant in any way to be insulting of cyclists, I think when a cyclist gets all geared up for his or her Saturday morning ride (with other cyclists), it is kind of like Halloween when you get to dress up and be somebody else for a day. I have seen quite a few otherwise mild mannered businessmen and women look pretty wild when decked out in cycling apparel. Still others like cycling because it can be a very social activity.

Patients with type 2 diabetes may like cycling for any of the above-mentioned reasons or because it has such a profound effect on lowering blood glucose levels and improving HbA1C scores. Although I would like to believe that everyone who exercises does it to improve or maintain their health and that everyone with diabetes does it to reduce insulin resistance, lose some fat and maintain good blood glucose control, that is simply not the case. There are all sorts of reasons people exercise and becoming healthier or improving blood glucose control is not always the primary goal.

Many people begin to exercise to lose weight, simply because they want to look better; perhaps by losing weight they believe they will be more accepted, gain friends, be more appealing to the opposite sex, etc. The improved health benefits that go along with the weight loss are secondary to them. As far as I am concerned, as long as people are exercising and deriving the results exercise has to offer, it doesn't really matter to me why they are exercising, I am just really glad they are.

In summation, it is first important to find an exercise that is do-able in light of possible cardiovascular and orthopedic constraints and equally important, an exercise that is in some way enjoyable or rewarding.

An ideal situation would be to find an aerobic exercise that you like and then add some resistance training (weight lifting) to that. Keep in mind that all weight lifting does not involve lifting dumbbells or barbells. If the idea of lifting dumbbells and barbells is not appealing and conjures up feelings of apprehension and pain, no problem, there are other options. Skip the dumbbells and barbells and use weight machines; they are easier and safer to use and accomplish the same results.

Frequency of Exercise

According to the previously listed Clinical Practice Guidelines, at least 150 minutes per week of moderate-intensity activity (50-70 percent of maximum heart rate) is recommended and/or at least 90 minutes per week of vigorous aerobic exercise (>70 percent of maximum heart rate). The physical activity should be spread out over at least three days per week and with no more than two consecutive days without physical activity. (47)

The U.S. Surgeon General's Report recommends that most people exercise for a minimum of 30 minutes on most, ideally all, days of the week. (50) As you can see, both reports are very similar in regards to the duration of exercise recommended, at least 30 minutes of exercise per session. They differ though in respect to the frequency of exercise. I prefer the Surgeon General's Report to the Clinical Practice guidelines as it recommends greater frequency. (50) Let me point out though that the Surgeon General's report is intended for the general population, not a specific population such as people with diabetes or other medical conditions. The ADA Clinical Practice Guidelines are specifically for people with diabetes and suggest three to five days per week of aerobic exercise (walking, cycling, swimming, water exercise, etc.) (52)

Although I have never collected data to support this observation, I am of the belief that, at least with my patients, the more often they exercise the better the result. I hypothesize this would be the case for all patients with type 2 diabetes. One study shows that even when exercise is performed as little as twice per week, patients see improvement in their diabetes control. (47) This is consistent with what I have observed in my patients. When they exercise less frequently, they still see improvement in blood glucose control, however, not as much improvement as when exercise is performed more frequently. Although blood glucose control has been shown to improve with twice a week exercise sessions, it is not likely to stimulate significant improvement in cardiovascular function. (56)

Generally speaking any exercise is better than no exercise. So even if a patient progresses from no exercise to minimal exercise, there are benefits. You don't want to be in the situation of only being able to exercise two times per week and saying, "What's the point, exercising twice a week is not enough to do me any good?" As I just mentioned, even though twice a week is not much exercise, it does produce results. Generally speaking, I do see less long-term benefits when patients exercise less often or infrequently. As for the patients I see in my office, those experiencing the greatest benefits are those exercising the most often, some at 5-7 days per week. Some patients even exercise on their own one or two days over the weekend, which for these patients means exercising daily or almost daily. It is interesting to note that those exercising at least one day over the weekend tend to have a much easier time exercising when they return for exercise on Monday. This is not only found to be true in patients with diabetes but for many people who exercise regularly. Could it be that, although not necessarily measurable, our bodies begin to decondition after just 48 hours of inactivity, making the return to exercise on Monday a little less comfortable than the exercise performed on the other days of the week?

There is no doubt in my mind that the more often patients with diabetes exercises, within reason of course, the better they will be able to control their diabetes. For those patients focused on weight loss as well as improved blood glucose control, it has been suggested to be physically active between five and seven days per week at lower intensity levels. (52,57) More research is needed that looks at the relationship between the volume of exercise performed and the benefits that result, specifically looking at how much exercise is required to realize maximum benefits and whether there is a point when further increasing exercise time yields diminishing returns.

Duration of Exercise

The patients I have been working with for the last six to seven years seem to have the best success when most of their exercise sessions last approximately one hour. On days when they are feeling really good they may exercise an hour and ten or an hour and twenty minutes. On days when they are not quite as energetic they may only exercise for 30 to 45 minutes.

Once one of my patients becomes comfortable with the exercise routine we have mutually agreed upon and has done it for a little while, I usually leave it up to the patient to decide how much to do based on how they are feeling that day. Exercise performed for less than an hour, such as 30–45 minutes can produce significant results. It has been my observation, however, that at least with the type 2 patients that I work with, even better results are achieved when the patient exercises closer to an hour. With the longer exercise time comes increased blood glucose utilization resulting in lower blood glucose levels and greater usage of stored energy, such as fat. Both are good things to see as long as the patients have the energy and their blood glucose level does not drop too low.

The previously mentioned clinical practice guidelines recommend at least 150 minutes per week of moderate intensity activity at 50-70 percent of maximal heart rate or at least 90 minutes per week of vigorous aerobic exercise at (>70 percent of maximum heart rate). (47)

As you can easily ascertain, you have the option of exercising more vigorously 3 times per week for 30 minutes or less vigorously 5 times per week for 30 minutes. In other words the more vigorously you exercise the less frequently you will need to exercise. Also, the more vigorously you exercise the faster you will use up energy, or more familiarly, "burn calories." Conversely, the lower the exercise intensity the longer it will take to burn calories.

Caloric utilization or energy expenditure can also be used to determine how frequently and how long to exercise. The American College of Sports Medicine recommends a caloric expenditure of 150-400 calories per day. (58) This amounts to a minimum caloric expenditure of 1000 calories per week, which is thought to be associated with a decrease in all cause mortality risk. (58) Certainly people who have not exercised in a while and are considered out of shape should start off near the 150 calorie per day goal and gradually progress toward the 400 calorie per day goal as their conditioning improves. A caloric expenditure of 2000 calories per week has been shown to contribute to the success of short and long-term weight loss. (58) I have preferred that many of my patients exercise more frequently but at a lower intensity because I believe they are at less risk of having a cardiovascular event (heart attack or stroke) at a lower intensity and that they will be more comfortable performing the exercise, improving the odds of them adhering to the exercise program long term.

Many patients are pleased to find out they can split up their exercise time throughout the day into two or three different sessions. Cardiorespiratory improvements have been found to be similar for those who exercise in short bouts of 10 minutes three times per day and those who exercise for approximately 30 minutes nonstop. (54,57)

This works out great for people who don't have time to do all of their exercise at one time, get too tired doing all of their exercise at one time, or get too bored doing all of their exercise at one time. The downside to breaking up the total exercise time into smaller segments is that research shows that 30 to 60 minutes of continuous exercise is more beneficial for weight loss. (52) For those not concerned with weight loss the only problem then is the need for more showers. You know, sweating and all.

In the past these patients might just skip the exercise altogether if they only had the time, energy or fortitude to exercise for only 15 minutes. One patient may choose to exercise for 45 minutes a day and divide it up into three 15 minute segments, one after breakfast, one after lunch and one after dinner, while another patient gets the same results exercising for 45 minutes at one time. It's really up to the person to do what works best. Ultimately, you will want to work it out any way you can in order to get the exercise in.

Intensity of Exercise

It seems like ever since we were very young we were led to believe that the harder we exercise the better the results. I also used to think that if I blew my nose really hard I wouldn't feel congested anymore and that drinking Grape Nehi cola would turn my insides purple. Well, that's not true and all blowing my nose really hard ever did was cause my sinus passages to swell making it even more difficult to breathe!

So what about the notion that the harder we exercise the better the result, is it true? Only to a point, and this is where many patients make mistakes and have problems. There are lots and lots of people, patients included, who have been told one too many times that the harder they work the better the results. In most cases though once a moderate level of exertion is reached, there is no reason to increase the intensity of the exercise beyond that. There are exceptions to this, however, and most of these exceptions concern competitive athletes. For an athlete to get in tiptop shape it is necessary for some workouts to be vigorous. These vigorous workouts are likely to be perceived as difficult or hard by the athlete. Unless participating in competitive sports or achieving a high level of cardiovascular fitness is the patient's goal, there is no reason to exercise vigorously.

I want to stress here that with very few exceptions people do not want to work so hard that they become significantly uncomfortable.

Exercising at an inappropriate intensity is probably responsible for a large majority of people not continuing with a fitness program long term. I truly believe that the saying, "no pain, no gain" has harmed far more people than it has ever helped, and it is unfortunate that the phrase ever caught on and had such an influence on how hard people exercised.

There are some very good reasons why patients with diabetes should consider moderate intensity exercise versus vigorous exercise. The first is that nearly all of the benefits we look to gain from performing regular exercise can be realized at moderate intensities that are far less likely to cause significant discomfort or pain. The second reason to avoid really strenuous exercise is because the higher the intensity at which someone exercises, the greater the risk of having some type of cardiac or circulatory problem develop during exercise, or in other words, a heart attack or stroke.

The third and fourth reason to avoid really strenuous exercise is that it generally is not comfortable and is unnecessary. If you can achieve most all of the same benefits from moderate intensity exercise as high intensity exercise and with much less discomfort, then why do the high intensity work? How likely would you be to continue with an exercise program if every time you exercised it hurt? That's what I thought. Me too!

Now, if you found that you were getting really great results by performing high intensity exercise you might be willing to put up with the discomfort short term, but odds are you wouldn't be willing to do it long term. Long-term compliance is the goal.

Fortunately, we now know that high intensity exercise is not necessary to get good results. Maybe people who were driven away from exercise because it was a pain will consider giving it another try if it's not likely to hurt. I sure hope so.

Exercise is simply too important to skip just because it may have been uncomfortable or produced some soreness in the past. We can do things to minimize or limit muscle soreness.

So how do you know just how hard you are exercising and whether it is too hard, or even, in many cases too easy. Remember that exercising too easily is not good either as you are not likely to maximize your results. Sometimes when patients come to me two or three months after starting the exercise program and say they have not seen much improvement, their lack of progress can be directly related to the amount of effort he or she has put into the exercise program.

All you really know now, assuming you agree with me, is that you don't want to work really hard like you would be doing with high intensity exercise; however, you do want to work hard enough to get results. Keep reading and in the next several pages you will find out how to determine jut how hard you are exercising.

Methods of Determining Exercise Intensity: There are a number of different methods for gauging how hard you are working during exercise. Some involve using your heart rate as a guide while others use simpler "exertion" scales posted on the wall. There are other methods where you exercise at a percentage of your VO2 max, (maximal oxygen uptake); however the determination of VO2 max usually requires some type of maximal exertion test and is either not readily available or not safe for many people.

The vast majority of people who want to measure or keep track of how vigorously they exercise do so by monitoring their heart rate during exercise and trying to keep it within a calculated heart rate range. There are two popular and widely used methods for doing this however, I must warn you that although popular and widely used, both methods have a major drawback and may not be safe for everyone to use. The method I will explain first is the easiest to use and for that reason may be why it is used more often. In fact if you have ever used a piece of exercise equipment with the words "target heart rate range" posted somewhere on the display, this is the method used to calculate those ranges.

Using Percentage of Maximal Heart Rate: The first step in this process is to calculate your estimated maximal heart rate by subtracting your age from 220. Depending on what shape you are in (or not in), you would then take this number and multiply it first by a percentage of 100. This will give you the lower limit of your heart rate range. You would then take the same number you started with but this time multiply it by a number that is ten percent higher than you did the first time. This will give you the upper limit of your target heart rate range. Typically, if you were not very fit you would want to select a relatively low range in which to start, something like 50-60 percent of maximal heart rate. As your fitness level improves you would then calculate a slightly higher percentage of your maximal heart rate at which to exercise. The premise here is that the higher the percentage of maximal heart rate at which you are able to exercise, the more aerobically fit you will become.

A similar method for measuring exercise intensity utilizes the Karvonen equation to calculate heart rate reserve (HRR). (59) The difference between this method and the previous method is that this method takes into consideration a person's resting heart rate. Resting heart rate can be one indication of a person's level of fitness. Many well-trained endurance athletes have resting heart rates as low as the high 30's. This is largely attributable to the athlete's heart being able to pump large quantities of blood each time it beats and the stimulation of nerves that actually slow the beat of the heart.

By taking resting heart rate into account a more individualized target heart rate range can be calculated. To do this, after subtracting your age from 220, then subtract your resting heart rate from that number. The resulting number is then multiplied as above, by a lower percentage and then again by a percentage ten percent higher. The resting heart rate is then added back to each number. These numbers will represent the lower and upper limits of the target heart rate range.

There is one major drawback to using both of these methods, however.

Without doing a maximal stress test under professionally supervised conditions, there is no way to accurately determine a person's maximal heart rate. The 220 minus age formula for determining maximal heart rate may predict values that are totally inaccurate, leading to patients exercising at heart rate levels that are either dangerously high or too low to significantly improve cardiovascular conditioning. In one study, it was stated that the idea of a formula to predict an individual's maximum heart rate is ludicrous. (60) Another study by the same author suggested that there was very little scientific basis for using this formula. (61)

In addition to this major drawback, there is yet another reason why using target heart rate formulas is not appropriate for a lot of people with diabetes. This is because if you take a medication in the class of drugs known as "beta blockers" or if you have autonomic neuropathy your heart rate is not going to respond, as it should with increasing levels of exertion. Beta-blockers typically keep the heart rate from climbing very high during exercise regardless of how hard you exercise and are designed to reduce the overall workload of the heart. If you don't understand this and keep increasing the exercise intensity in order to get the heart rate into your target heart rate range and the heart rate fails to climb as it should it could be very dangerous. This may cause you to exercise at a much higher intensity than is safe for your age, overall health status, etc. People taking beta -blockers should not use exercise heart rates as a means for prescribing or measuring exercise intensity.

If a person has autonomic neuropathy (AN), physiological adjustments that should automatically occur, either don't work or don't work well. As an example, for the person without (AN), heart rate and blood pressure would both increase in a somewhat predicted manner with increasing exercise intensity. For people diagnosed or suspected of having (AN) it is entirely possible that neither heart rate nor blood pressure would respond normally to exercise. Therefore, people with diabetes that are known to have or suspected of having (AN), should use an alternate form of measuring exercise intensity and forgo using a percentage of maximum heart rate.

If you decide to use either of the methods I have just described, a percentage of maximum heart rate or the HRR method, be aware that the calculated target heart rate range should only be used as a guide. If you find that exercising in your target heart rate range is unpleasant and seems to be too much of an exertion, then don't do it, back off a bit.

That particular heart rate range may be just a bit too high, for now. It doesn't mean you will never be comfortable exercising at this intensity, but for now you are, so I recommend you don't do it. If you want to continue using exercise heart rates as a means of measuring your exercise intensity, I suggest you lower the range by ten percent, maybe exercising at that intensity will work better for you, for now. Granted, the cardiovascular conditioning may not occur as fast or to the same degree when exercising at a lower intensity; however, if you continue to exercise at an intensity that is too uncomfortable or that keeps you in a constant state of soreness, then you are probably not going to continue your exercise regimen for very long. Think about this for a minute, if you consider the 30 minute walk you do in the morning the longest 30 minutes of the day, how long do you think you are going to stick with it?

What good is it going to do to get your heart rate within the target heart rate range if within a week or two or three you are going to quit walking altogether because it hurts too much, or because you just consider it too difficult?

It's going to do very little good, if any, because the exercise routine was so short lived.

This kind of thing happens all the time. People start an exercise program after reading guidelines or hearing from people about how they need to get their heart rates up to a certain level in order to lose fat or burn any calories or to, basically, get any results. Then they go out and try it, find it uncomfortable to work that hard, but stick it out for a short time until they say forget this. Unfortunately, there is a lot of misinformation out there regarding exercise, and listening to the wrong advice can ruin your exercise program.

In summary, if target heart rate range is to be used to gauge exercise intensity, it should be done in combination with perceived exertion. If you are exercising in your calculated "target heart rate" range but feel that your level of exertion is too high, then the target heart rate range should be reduced to a range that is more comfortable. Remember if it's too uncomfortable you're not likely to make exercise a regular part of your life.

This brings me to the method of measuring exercise intensity with which I have had the most success.

Ratings of Perceived Exertion: In order for exercise to be of benefit to people with diabetes, it needs to be done on a regular basis, for a reasonable amount of time, and over the long term. It's not so much about getting someone to start exercising; it's more about getting them to continue exercising for the months and years to come. The best way I have found to increase that likelihood is to make sure that patients exercise well within their capabilities so as not to produce pain or any significant discomfort. When monitoring patients who exercise in my office, I am always looking for signs that indicate the patient is working too hard or even too easy.

Generally speaking, I like for my patients to gradually increase their exercise intensity level to a point just shy of causing any significant discomfort. When patients ask me if they are working hard enough, I ask them how they feel. The answer to that question usually tells me everything I need to know to answer their question. In most cases I don't need to know what their heart rate is or even their blood pressure, just how they feel. Remember, if the patient has autonomic neuropathy or takes beta-blockers, the heart rate and blood pressure response to exercise is likely to be altered and a poor indication of how hard the patient is exercising.

For the just discussed reasons, I prefer to use Borg's Ratings of Perceived Exertion scale as one of two methods I use to prescribe exercise intensity. Named after the man who developed it, Gunnar Borg, the Ratings of Perceived Exertion scale, or RPE scale, is used to subjectively indicate how much effort is put into the exercise. (62)

As an example, if I suggest to patients that they exercise at a level 13 on the 6-20 scale and they are familiar with the use of the scale, then they know exactly how hard I want them to work. Similarly, if I ask patients how hard they are working, and they tell me 9 on the 6-20 scale, I know exactly how hard they are working. There are actually two scales, the original scale that goes from 6-20 and the revised scale that goes from 0-10. With each scale there is a descriptive word or words that correspond to most of the numbers. For example, on the 6-20 scale the words "very, very light" corresponds with the number 7. The descriptive by the number 9 is "very light." As the numbers go higher, the number 13 is described as "somewhat hard." The descriptive at 15 reads "hard," and 19 represents "very, very hard." (62)

Although the 6-20 scale works very well, the revised 0-10 may actually be used more frequently. The 0-10 scale is referred to as the modified Borg Scale. In my experiences, having used both scales, I believe one works as well as the other. I don't think it makes much difference which scale is used as long as the patient understands how to properly use the scale.

Table 5 - Rating of Perceived Exertion Scales

Original Rating Scale	New Rating Scale
6	0 Nothing at all
7 Very, very light	0.5 Very, very light (just noticeable)
8	
9 Very light	1 Very light
10	
11 Fairly light	2 Light (weak)
12	3 Moderate
13 Somewhat hard	4 Somewhat hard
14	
15 Hard	5 Heavy (strong)

16	6
17 Very hard	7 Very hard
18	8
19 Very, very hard	9
20	10 Very, very heavy (almost max

Borg, G.A.V. Reprinted with permission

In my facility, I have chosen to modify the scale even further. I use the 0-10 scale and have changed the descriptive very slightly. Wherever the word "light" appears I have substituted the word "easy". I have found that many of my patients can describe their effort more accurately by making this slight substitution.

When a patient is exercising in an exercise facility and these scales are posted, I highly recommend using them. When the patient is out doors walking or jogging or swimming or biking and obviously cannot see the scale, or when I am discussing exercise intensity in class, I recommend an even simpler scale that anybody can use at any time. A 1-10 scale, a scale you have probably used on many occasions. A scale you have used to rate how good something tasted or how attractive or handsome someone was. As an example, "The winner of the Miss America pageant was gorgeous. I would give her a 9 1/2 out of 10." Or "Well, considering we missed our plane, slept in the airport, got stung by a jellyfish and lost in the Grand Canyon, I would have to say our vacation was a disaster. I'd give it a 1 on a 1-10 scale. This scale is also used in hospitals to assess a patient's pain.

When I use the scale with patients, I explain it like this: on a scale of 1-10, 1 being no more effort than if you were lying down and 10 representing a maximal effort, I recommend that you exercise at a 5. This of course puts you right in the middle between really hard and really easy. I would call this a moderate pace. You should feel like you are definitely doing something but not really working hard enough to be uncomfortable. You should be breathing deeper and faster and you should notice your heart beating faster but definitely not racing.

This moderate but comfortable pace is fast enough to do most of the things we need exercise to do. It won't get you in racing shape but is good enough to contribute significantly to weight loss, reduce insulin resistance, increase insulin sensitivity, and help lower cardiac risk factors such as total cholesterol, LDL cholesterol, triglycerides and blood pressure. HDL cholesterol levels should rise as well. If you are feeling really good and want to improve your cardiovascular system a little more, you could push it a little harder and go up to a 6 on the scale. This would be considered a little harder than moderate exertion, and it may be a bit tougher to talk while exercising, although labored talking should still be possible. As for the patients really trying to maximize the cardiovascular benefits exercise has to offer, the intensity may be bumped up to a 7. Keep in mind though that at a seven, on the 1-10 scale, you would be working fairly hard, probably hard enough to cause some discomfort and harder than I recommend for most of my patients, particularly those with complications. I usually discourage going any higher than a seven on the scale for any of my patients for two major reasons.

The first reason is that although the long term benefits of exercise are numerous and substantial and reduce the risk of having a heart attack or stroke, there is also an increased risk of having a cardiac event (heart attack or stroke), while actually performing the exercise. So, generally speaking, the higher the exercise intensity, the greater the risk of a cardiac event while doing the exercise. My thinking is that if the benefits of exercise begin to diminish once a certain level of effort or intensity is put forth and the risks of injury continue to climb beyond that point, then the intensity should be increased no further.

The second reason is that higher intensity exercise is usually accompanied with a greater degree of discomfort. As mentioned previously, performing exercise should not produce any significant discomfort. If you knew that every time you exercised it was going to be painful or uncomfortable, you would start finding reasons to miss or delay your daily workouts.

One remaining method that I like for measuring exercise intensity is the "talk test." I tell patients that if you and someone else are out walking and you are walking so fast that you become too winded to talk, then slow down. If on the other hand you are walking so slowly you find yourself whistling or singing to your partner, then speed up. You are walking way too slow. The talk test works great in most situations, not swimming, though; I'm sure you can see why.

I really like recommending the talk test because it is so easy to use and it works so well.

In fact about a year ago I used the talk test personally, or actually, the principle behind the talk test, and it worked wonderfully.

Every Friday afternoon about three or four of my running friends and I would meet after work and go for our weekly group run. Now these were all good friends of mine, and I enjoyed their company, usually. But you know sometimes, not real often, but sometimes, for any number of reasons, there are days when you just don't want to be there. You would rather forgo the run or bike ride or swim and just go home and have a good dinner. Well, at least that is the way it was for me. But I couldn't, and I didn't have a good excuse to tell my friends to get out of the run. They could sense a phony excuse a mile away and be quite intimidating. They could be a pretty tough bunch. Anyway, with no excuse, and no threat of rain and lightning, I had no choice but to put my shorts and shoes on run. My strategy; just stay with the group, keep to yourself and get it over with, next week will be better.

Well we take off, and not more than 200 yards into the run somebody starts with the jokes. Why is it that whenever I just want to get it over with, everybody else is feeling chipper? Then the jokes keep coming, one after another. I'm thinking I can't do this for an hour. This has got to stop. So, I would pick up my pace a little. The jokes temporarily subsided, at least until everyone adapted to the new pace. Then the jokes returned. Not fast enough I guess. So I picked up my pace a little more. Once again, there was a temporary silence. Some of the guys quit talking altogether. It had become too difficult to talk and run. A few moments later one of my friends who was still able to talk commented that I must not have liked the jokes.

For the remainder of the run, with the exception of the water stops, it was quiet. It had become too difficult for us to talk and run at the same time. A run that typically took about an hour we finished in about 50 minutes. After the run the laughter and conversation returned. It didn't bother me then, the run was over, I felt a whole lot better and less stressed and could now go home and eat dinner. Now, that was my story, I do not recommend that you do what I did. For most people I recommend t they slow their pace and lower the exercise intensity when talking becomes too laborious.

In the last several pages I have tried to make clear the exercise guidelines established by the various professional and governmental agencies in regards to type 2 diabetes. To get the best possible results from exercise it is important to try and follow the guidelines mentioned above. The more closely these guidelines are followed, the more likely exercise will do what you need for it to do, improve insulin resistance and overall diabetes control, help protect and strengthen the cardiovascular and respiratory system and increase muscle strength and endurance.

Precautions

1. Always let your doctors know that you plan to start exercising. Even though exercise is so very important and can have such a tremendous impact on improving diabetes control, there are unfortunately some people who should not exercise. These people usually have one or more co-morbid conditions (a co-morbid condition is another serious medical problem), and as a result, the exertion that comes with exercise might exacerbate the condition. Sometimes patients with co-morbid conditions can still exercise as long as they are willing to modify some aspect of the exercise prescription. You will see examples of this as I continue. Regardless of whether there are co-morbid conditions present, anyone with diabetes should discuss exercise plans with their doctor before embarking on an exercise program. **Remember that with the diagnosis of diabetes comes the increased risk of having heart disease or stroke. This underscores the importance of having a check up with your doctor prior initiating exercise.** Your doctor can then decide if it is safe to initiate an exercise program or if some tests may need to be performed first to help ensure your safety.

2. Always check your blood glucose levels before and after exercise. This will help ensure that your blood glucose levels are sufficiently high at the start of exercise to provide a cushion to allow them some room to drop without the concern that they will drop too low. By too low I mean to levels low enough to produce hypoglycemic (low blood glucose) symptoms.

Blood glucose levels are likely to drop more drastically and to lower levels in people who take a medication that either stimulates the production and release of insulin by the beta cells or people who inject insulin. Consequently, for these people, it is very important to check blood glucose levels before initiating the exercise.

As an example, for people taking medications stimulating insulin production or taking insulin injections, typically the appearance of hypoglycemic symptoms becomes evident when blood glucose levels drop as low as 75 or 80mg/dl. It is important for these people to know that the blood glucose levels at which hypoglycemic symptoms appear one day may be different than the levels at which they appear on another day. Knowing that hypoglycemia may occur at levels somewhere around 75-80mg/dl., these people would be wise to make sure their blood glucose levels are sufficiently high to allow for a substantial drop in blood glucose during exercise with their levels still being above that which causes hypoglycemia.

Determining how much blood glucose levels will drop during and immediately following exercise is not something that can be calculated. A rough estimate is about the best you can do and sometimes that is way off. One day walking a mile at 3 mph may lower blood glucose levels 85mg/dl.,while the next day doing the exact same thing under what seems to be the exact same circumstances might lower the blood glucose level 45mg/dl.

The point I want to make here is that you can never predict with certainty how much your blood glucose level may drop as a result of performing exercise. Possibly the biggest reason for this is because even though conditions may appear to be identical from one exercise session to another, they are never identical. There are too many variables, many that we often don't even think about or that are not obvious, that influence the effect exercise has on blood glucose levels.

For the best protection against an unforeseen hypoglycemic episode, check blood glucose levels before exercise, and if below approximately 120mg/dl., take a small snack such as 4 ounces of juice or a small piece of fruit. This should boost blood glucose levels approximately 50-60mg/dl., enough so that if exercise caused a drop in blood glucose of that much or maybe a little more hypoglycemia would not result.

As an example, if you were going to drive from Miami Beach to Jacksonville in a big SUV that got very poor gas mileage and when you got in the car you noticed the gas gauge was sitting on a quarter of a tank, could you make it to Jacksonville? No, because you wouldn't have enough gas. Would you cancel the trip? No, you would go get some gas. How much? Enough to get you where you needed to go which in this case is Jacksonville. Similarly, if you find the blood glucose level is not high enough to safely permit you to do the exercise you want to do without fear of your blood glucose going too low, then you add some sugar to your blood by eating a small snack, raising your blood glucose level sufficiently, and thus allowing you to exercise safely.

Although the most significant drop in blood glucose is likely to occur during the actual exercise itself, it frequently happens that blood glucose levels continue to drop at an accelerated rate even after the exercise is completed. In some instances, blood glucose levels continue to drop at an accelerated rate for 30-60 minutes or so after the exercise, whereas on other occasions, the rate at which the blood glucose level drop, slows dramatically upon finishing the exercise. In still other cases, the blood glucose may drop somewhat during exercise, appear to stop dropping at the completion of exercise, and then drop considerably several hours after the completion of exercise. This is called delayed onset hypoglycemia and can be quite problematic. This delayed and often dramatic drop in blood glucose levels can result in hypoglycemic episodes occurring in the car on the way to work, while sitting in important meetings, in the middle of the night, or just about anytime during the day or night.

For this reason it is wise to also check blood glucose levels after exercise as well as before. By doing this, if the post exercise blood glucose level is anywhere close to the level at which hypoglycemia occurs, a light snack should be taken. As an example if hypoglycemia frequently occurs when blood glucose levels approach 75 or 80mg/dl. and post exercise blood glucose levels are close to 100mg/dl. or definitely below 100mg/dl., and the next meal is not immediately forthcoming, it would be very prudent to have a light snack. This snack should protect the patient if blood glucose levels were to continue dropping or if there was a delayed drop.

It is always a good idea for patients on diabetes medication, that is, those medications that stimulate the release of insulin from the beta cells or those requiring insulin injections, to keep a treatment with them at all times. That way it can be taken in the event of an unforeseen hypoglycemic episode. This could consist of a roll of lifesavers, several pieces of hard candy, or a small box of raisins. Glucose tablets or glucose gel are specifically designed for this use and can be purchased at most pharmacies.

For patients not taking medications that stimulate the release of insulin from the beta cells or not administering subcutaneous insulin, it is still recommended to check blood glucose levels before and after exercise. This is because it is still possible for blood glucose levels to drop too low, although it is not likely to happen. Another benefit of checking blood glucose levels pre and post exercise is that it can be very motivating for the patient. It is great motivation for a patient to exercise when they see how their blood glucose levels can drop substantially with only 30-45 minutes of exercise.

For patients not taking any diabetes medication, blood glucose levels are still going to drop with exercise, however, probably not to hypoglycemic producing levels.

3. People with significant neuropathy should avoid weight-bearing exercise. This is of extreme importance, particularly if there is some degree of numbness in the feet.

Careful consideration should always be given to which exercise or exercises are selected, based on present physical problems or complications. As an example, for someone with moderate to severe neuropathy in the feet and/or legs a weight bearing exercise such as walking, stair climbing, step aerobics or using an elliptical machine would be contraindicated, not a good idea.

Remember that neuropathy is nerve damage that can cause significant pain in the feet and may ultimately lead to total numbness in one or both feet. When feeling is lost in the foot, or feet, as the case may be, patients may change the way they walk, putting their feet down differently from usual. This can result in undue stress being applied to parts of the feet not designed to handle that degree of stress. This can lead to tissue breakdown and eventually ulcerations, which can prove very difficult to heal.

A better choice for the patient with neuropathy would be a non-weight bearing exercise like cycling or swimming. Swimming of course should be avoided if there are open wounds anywhere on the body due to risk of infection. Non-weight bearing exercise keeps the weight off of the patient's legs and feet, which is what you want to do.

Also, if a patient has joint problems, particularly in the low back, hips, knees and feet, a non-weight bearing exercise may be more appropriate such as cycling or swimming. Water exercise is an alternative to swimming if multiple joint problems limit a patient's ability to swim. A strong word of caution here: If a patient cannot swim, they are not safe in the water and should not be in a pool. The way I look at it, if a patient ends up drowning in a pool, what's the point in preventing long-term complications?

Ultimately, stationary cycling may end up being the exercise of choice for a large majority of the people with peripheral neuropathy. I tend to recommend stationary cycling over outdoor cycling if there are any balance concerns and the patient for any number of reasons seems to be at an increased risk of falling.

4. Do not exercise if sick.

This puts an increased strain on the body and increases the work the heart has to do. It may also delay getting over the illness.

5. Do not exercise right after eating.

There is a significant increase in the amount of blood that goes to the stomach right after eating. It has been estimated that 70% of a person's total blood volume is involved in the digestive process right after eating. This means there is less blood available for the muscles to use during exercise. The heart and vascular system will try to make adaptations to supply the working muscles with adequate quantities of blood; however, this puts an unnecessary strain on the heart. It is therefore recommended to wait approximately an hour after eating before starting to exercise. As a rule of thumb, the larger the meal, or the greater the quantity of fat in the meal, the longer you should wait before exercising. You would be wise to postpone your exercise when feeling "stuffed" or "full."

6. Keep an emergency treatment for hypoglycemia with you at all times.

In the event blood glucose levels unexpectedly drop to levels that are too low, it is recommended that all patients with diabetes keep a hypoglycemic treatment with them at all times. Glucose tablets or glucose gel (available at most pharmacies) are both good choices as well as a roll of lifesavers or several pieces of hard candy.

7. Begin each exercise session slowly.

No matter how fit you are, or become, begin each exercise session slowly and gradually increase the pace until you reach the desired pace. This allows time for capillaries and larger blood vessels to deliver blood to the areas where it is needed.

8. End each exercise session slowly.

Whatever exercise is being performed, always slow down gradually over the last approximately 5minutes. This reduces the occurrence of feeling lightheaded, dizzy or generally feeling queasy when the exercise is complete. The practice of warming down or "cooling" down towards the end of the exercise session helps blood that was shifted away from non-exercising muscles to exercising muscles to shift back again.

9. Don't overdo it.

It might sound unlikely that a patient would do this, particularly one who does not like to exercise to begin with, but it does. What sometimes happens in these cases is that patients start seeing such good results from the exercise that they are motivated to exercise even more. Exercise duration that initially was 15 to 20 minutes once per day has now been increased to what is now 1½ -2 hours twice per day! Although likely to produce good results, the exercise has become a bit excessive and it is not likely, because of the time and effort involved, that the patient will continue with it long term. I have seen this kind of thing happen many, many times. It is simply not reasonable to expect that most people will continue with an exercise regimen that is so time consuming regardless of the great results they are seeing. The beginning of the end usually starts when the patient realizes that this amount of exercise or time to do the exercise cannot continue. This leads to a reduction in the exercise so that he or she is now exercising an hour per day. After having exercised for up to three to four hours recently, an hour of exercise doesn't seem like much anymore and similarly doesn't seem worth doing to a lot of people. The satisfaction of doing a lot of exercise is lost and before you know it the patient starts missing exercise sessions;

"things come up". It's not usually long after this that so many things "come up" that performing an hour of exercise each day becomes less and less frequent, until eventually the patient has stopped exercising altogether.

I have seen this so many times with my patients that when I notice a patient continuing to bump up their exercise time and the time they stay in the facility too much over an hour, I pull them aside and discuss the pitfalls that may result. I remind them of the story of the tortoise and the hare; how slow and steady wins the race. It is consistent, moderately paced exercise that tends to provide the best results. That being said, a patient, or anyone for that matter that totally exhausts him or herself during exercise either by working too vigorously or for too long is definitely overdoing it. With the possible exception of competitive athletes, it is of absolutely no benefit for anyone to do so much exercise that they are exhausted when finished. It may actually be quite harmful as it also increases the likelihood of burnout similar to the way exercising too long does.

Just think about it. If you thought it was necessary to exhaust yourself when you worked out, for whatever reason, considering the practicality of doing such a thing and the associated discomfort then and later, do you think you would continue to exercise long term? Not likely, at least not if you are like most people.

What If You Do Not Like to Exercise?

I have heard of this happening. Perhaps even some of you reading this book may have at one time or another had some unkind words to say about exercise.

"I don't like to do any exercise. I never have. I don't even like to sweat!"

Or you may be thinking, "When am I going to find the time to exercise? I don't even have the time to get the things done that I have to do now?" By the way, I'm not trying to make life more difficult for you, but exercise is one of those things that needs to be added to that list of things you have to do but don't have time for.

Not having time to exercise is an obstacle for a lot of people who otherwise would like to exercise. There is certainly no shortage of obstacles getting in the way. Regardless of the number of obstacles, the importance of exercise doesn't change. I won't downplay its significance or disregard it because you don't like to do it or because it's really hard to squeeze into an already busy day. You simply need to work harder at figuring out a way to make exercise more palatable if you don't like to do it and a way to overcome the many obstacles that get in the way of exercise if that's the problem.

Granted, some patients have only a few obstacles to overcome; some are going to have to work harder than others to figure out what exercise they can do and when they can do it. Imagine for a moment that you give up on exercise because it's just too much of a hassle overcoming the obstacles. Let's assume your diabetes control gets worse, complications set in, you cope with them the best you can, for a while, but eventually you have to move on, like to heaven. One afternoon you are sitting around, casually chatting with others about your children and grandchildren still living and how you miss them. One of the ladies, a female spirit that is, asks you, "What happened, what brought you up here?" "Diabetes complications," you answer.

"You didn't exercise?" she asks.

"No, I couldn't. I was just too busy. There was simply no time left to exercise after feeding the homeless in the morning, volunteering at the humane society in the afternoon and making dinner for lost animals in the evening. As you can see, with a schedule like that, there were good reasons why I couldn't get my exercise in," you explain.

"Good reasons or bad reasons, does it really make any difference? The fact remains that you are up here in heaven and your family is down there without you. Does having good reasons or bad reasons not to exercise make that any less painful?" Anyone can come up with excuses not to do something they don't want to do; after all, it takes no special skills or talent and very little effort. In fact, it has been rumored that the next easiest thing to do besides lying in bed doing nothing is making excuses about lying in bed doing nothing.

The moral of the story is don't make excuses overcome obstacles. Control your diabetes.

Don't give up. When you have type 2 diabetes, you cannot afford to give up, not on the most significant treatment there is for the disease. Giving up on exercise because you may not have had success in the past is like taking one of your medications and throwing it out the window because you often forget to take it anyway. You wouldn't do that would you? Now, if you just said, "No, of course not", then you are on the right track so please continue. If you said, "Yes, that sounds like something that I would do," I am not sure I can help you, go back to page 1.

For those of you who may not be so keen on exercise, or to put another way, you haven't really enjoyed any exercise you have tried in the past, we are going to assume you haven't tried the right one yet, the one that is best suited to your personality and lifestyle.

This is what I recommend to my patients. First you need to find someone who's willing to work with you on this, maybe your best friend or a colleague at work. Your mission: Find an exercise you like. I mean it. There is at least one out there. You just have to find it! Each week you and your buddy commit to trying a different exercise until you settle on an exercise you like. I'm not kidding. Don't limit yourself. Try anything and everything you can as long as it is safe. Make it an adventure. If you are doing this with a friend, the whole experience should be a lot of fun. Dance classes such as belly dancing, ballroom dancing and ballet are all good choices. Rock climbing, martial arts and fencing are other options you may not have thought about. Joining a softball league, a running club or a masters (adult) swim team would all allow you to get your exercise while being with others.

You may have to try a new activity every week or you may need a few weeks or longer to decide whether you like an activity enough to stick with it long term. Make a pact with your partner not to quit looking until you find an activity you like. Don't be surprised if you end up doing an activity or exercise you never in a million years thought you would be doing.

Please keep in mind the following:

Have you ever met someone that you didn't particularly like at first but are now good friends with? The same could be true for a particular exercise. Allow time for the exercise to grow on you. I am doubtful there are many activities you might try for the first time where you would say, "Wow, what a great exercise, I want to do that every day for at least 45 minutes!" If you try an activity only once or twice and make a decision as to whether you like it based only on those two trials alone is not really giving the activity a fair chance. Patients frequently ask me, "So what is the best exercise?" The answer I give them is always the same," I'll say it again, whatever exercise they like the most or whatever exercise they are most likely to do. It would be ludicrous for me to recommend an exercise to a patient that they have an aversion to. In a sense I would be contributing to their failure.

Suggestions to Help You Stick with It

Try disguising your exercise. One cool night, quite a few years ago when I was attending graduate school, I was walking from my car to my classroom and happened to walk past the basketball courts.

I wasn't paying a lot of attention but did notice about a dozen guys playing basketball. Several hours later as I was walking back to my car after class, I noticed that about twice as many guys were playing basketball. As I watched the players run back and forth up and down the court I realized that some of the guys playing now were guys that were playing several hours ago when I was on my way to class. These guys had been playing basketball for over two hours? Why do you think these guys were playing for so long?

Do you think it is because they needed the exercise? Not likely. Do you think it is because they really like basketball? Probably. If I ran over and stopped one of the players that had been playing all this time and asked him, "Did you realize you just got two hours of good high quality exercise while you were playing basketball?"

The player might shrug off the question and say, "Hey, I'm just playing basketball because I like basketball." This is what I call disguising exercise. The player was playing basketball because he likes basketball, not because he wanted to get two hours of exercise in. As it turned out not only did he have a lot of fun playing basketball but also got two hours of good high quality exercise at the same time.

Kids don't join soccer leagues because they want to get exercise but because they like playing soccer. Kids don't ride bikes to get exercise but because they like riding bikes. Teenagers don't do tricks and ride skateboards to get exercise but because they like skateboards. All of these activities are disguised exercises. If you could get involved in a hobby that happened to be active and that you really liked, that would be your best bet.

Get a buddy or two. Get someone to exercise with you. This would be someone you would be accountable to if you decided to skip your exercise one day.

When I was much younger, long ago, I was a competitive runner. This meant I needed to run on most days of the week. Now, I am probably not a lot different than you in that there were many mornings I just did not want to get out of bed at 5:45 a.m. and go run. On those mornings if I didn't have someone waiting for me on the other end of town at 6:30 a.m., I would have probably rolled over and gone back to sleep, even though I usually like to exercise (just not that early).

You notice how I said "usually". There are occasionally days when, no matter what time of day it is, I don't want to do any exercise at all. Every body has days like this. That's when it is good to have someone you are accountable to, someone depending on you to exercise with them. This strategy can help get you through your less motivated days and keep you on track.

Take a sedentary activity and make it active. Perhaps you could take a hobby or activity you already do now and make it active. For example, let's say that you have a friend that you talk with on the phone several mornings a week for 30-40 minutes after the kids get off to school. You suggest to your friend, who only lives several miles away, that he/she meet you at a specified location and you could walk while you talk. Maybe another day or two of the week or perhaps one day on the weekend you could meet with another friend and ride bikes while you talk.

Get a dog. It has been suggested that everyone with diabetes should have a dog and if they don't have one should get one. This would give you a reason to get out and walk. After all, you don't want your dog to develop diabetes. Every dog I have ever known loves to go for walks. Usually two or three per day, perfect! In order to get the most out of this strategy, however, there are a few simple guidelines you should be aware of. First of all get a dog with some legs on him, or her if you choose a female. What I mean by that is that if you get a dog that has legs no longer than 6-8 inches then you are going to have to walk pretty slow, thus limiting how far you can walk, how much sugar you can burn up and how much exercise your heart gets. I generally recommend a species with legs at least 15 inches from toenail to trunk. And finally try to avoid a frequent sniffer.

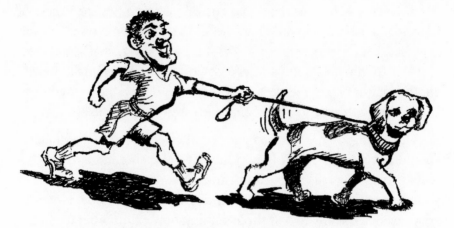

I do honestly believe that for the majority of people with type 2 diabetes, performing regular exercise is the most important treatment in managing the disease. To summarize, primarily because of its direct effect on decreasing insulin resistance as well as reducing body fat mass and helping control most of the major cardiovascular risk factors. It is for these reasons I place more emphasis on exercise than I do making changes in nutritional habits.

I will point out that I said for the majority of patients with type2 diabetes exercise is likely to be the most important and underutilized treatment. Of course there are those patients who have such poor eating habits that for them the adherence to an improved eating plan might be the first priority and fastest way to achieve better blood sugar control with increased physical activity taking a back seat, at least initially.

For some patients recommending they make too many changes in their lives at one time, such as eating better, starting to exercise and checking blood sugar levels can seem overwhelming. In these cases the treatment or skills thought necessary to provide the fastest and most extreme improvement in the patient's blood sugar control are prioritized and will be emphasized first. On the other hand many patients would prefer to go ahead and try to make several changes at one time. This is a perfect example of why there needs to be some degree of individualization in diabetes instruction. Depending on the needs of the patient, some aspects of treatment may need to be emphasized more than others.

Patient Comments Concerning Exercise

As a diabetes educator I have heard many interesting comments and stories from patients concerning exercise. I want to take a few moments here and share some of them and in some cases add comments of my own.

1. One day in class I had spent close to an hour building my case as to why I believed exercise may be the most important treatment for diabetes. When I finally came out and said it, that exercise might be the most important treatment for diabetes, a female patient sitting right in front of me who looked to be in her forties shook her head and stated, "I didn't exercise when I was younger, and I sure don't plan on starting now."

2. Another day we were in the midst of discussing the merits of exercise when a patient spoke up and said that exercise made her tired. I shifted my attention to the patient's comment and started to explore the reasons for her tiredness. Perhaps she was pushing herself too hard or not getting enough rest between exercise sessions. I hadn't gotten very far with the list of possibilities when the patient interrupted yet again remarking, "You know I am in my fifties!" Her inference was that it was somewhat expected to be tired when you are up in years like your fifties. It never occurred to her that it was very possible, even likely, that part of her reason for being tired and having little energy was due to a lack of exercise.

3. More recently, as I was beginning my discussion on exercise guidelines one morning, I mentioned that walking was an excellent exercise. As I continued discussing the benefits of walking I noticed that a patient started shaking her head as if to say no and was starting to smile. I looked at her and asked why are you shaking your head?

She responded, "Can't do it?"

"Can't do what?" I asked.

"Can't walk," she replied.

"Ok, how come?" I asked.

"It hurts my legs too bad. If I try to walk, I have to stop and quit after five minutes cause my legs hurt so bad," she answered.

"You might want to try walking somewhere like a mall where once your legs start hurting you can sit down and rest until they start to feel better. Then you can get up and walk a little bit more until they begin to hurt again. When that happens sit down and rest some more," I suggested.

Again, the patient starts shaking her head as if to say no and the smile appears. "Can't do it," she says.

"You don't think that might work?" I asked.

"There are too many smells in the mall and it bothers my asthma."

"Well it doesn't have to be a mall, any place where you have the opportunity to stop and rest periodically will do. How about swimming or water exercise, those are both good, particularly swimming?"

Again the patient starts shaking her head. "I can't do that either, I don't have a pool."

"Do you have access to a public pool?" I asked.

She shook her head no, while smiling.

"Okay," I said, "How about riding a stationary bike, that works for a lot of people and is a great exercise?"

Yet again she smiled and shook her head. At this point one thing was certain, that the patient could shake her head very well from side to side. If no other exercise worked I knew I could fall back on that one. "Why can't you ride a stationary bike?" I asked.

"I have hemorrhoids and it's just too painful," she stated.

I began to get the feeling this was all a game to her. It looked as though she was going to come up with an excuse to avoid doing anything I recommended. It wasn't funny, not to me anyway. It was actually sad. By now every time I suggested something the rest of the class looked at this lady to see if she was going to shake her head.

The patient, I believe, had pretty much convinced herself that she could not do any exercise due to her bad legs, asthma, hemorrhoids, etc. I think the patient thought she had some legitimate excuses not to exercise and whatever the consequences that resulted could not be helped. I couldn't let the patient leave class that day with that attitude. I had to at least try and change the way she felt about her ability to get some exercise.

After pausing a moment, trying to figure out how I could be the most effective, I walked over to the table where the patient was sitting and explained politely but firmly, "You have just got to move. You have got to figure out a way to move more than you have been. The more you move, the better your diabetes is likely to be. Granted it may be more difficult for you to become active, and you may have more obstacles to overcome than some other people you know, but remaining sedentary is not an option. That is, not if you want to improve your diabetes control and reduce your risks of developing complications in the future."

The patient wasn't shaking her head anymore and the smile was gone. With the patient now realizing that having some physical limitations does not necessarily preclude exercise, I hope the patient was trying to think of some activities she could still do instead of coming up with excuses for her recent inactivity. After all, I bet every single patient in my class that day could come up with an excuse not to exercise. Anybody can come up with excuses for something they don't want to do. That's not hard. But coming up with solutions to problems of course is more challenging.

One of the staff members I used to work with gave me a ride to work one day when my car was being repaired. I thought she was driving a bit fast and not as carefully as she should, as I kept having to hold onto the door handle with my right hand and brace my left hand on the center console just to stay in my seat. I suggested she slow down some.

Her response was, "We are running late and I thought you wanted to get to work on time." I told her I do want to get to work on time, but alive, and we may not make it to work at all if you keep driving like this. She said she was sorry and that she would slow down and again explained that she had been driving fast so we would not be late.

"Listen, if we get killed in a car accident, and I'm not around anymore, it is not going to make it excusable or any easier for my wife and kids to accept the fact that I am dead just because "we were trying not to be late to work."

To me the same is true with diabetes, exercise and complications. If a patient says he or she can't exercise due to a bad back, or knees or feet, etc., and this lack of exercise contributes to his or her development of complications and a reduced quality of life, are the complications going to be any less bothersome or acceptable to live with because the patient believes he or she had a good excuse for not exercising?

Orthopedic, cardiovascular or other limitations do not usually preclude exercise; it simply means they have to be more creative to figure out what they can do. In most cases, exercise is still possible, is strongly encouraged and is extremely beneficial.

4. My next to last story, for now, is of a thin man who sat in the back of my class one day and throughout a good portion of my exercise presentation made inappropriate comments about exercise and his need for it. After the exercise lecture the patients were taken to the cardiac rehabilitation office and given the opportunity to exercise for 10-20 minutes.

The purpose for doing this was to show the patients just how much their blood sugar levels dropped as a result of exercise, checking the patients' blood sugar levels before and after they exercised and observing the difference accomplished this.

The thin man spoke up towards the end of my lecture and explained that he got all of the exercise he needed at work. When I asked the patient what kind of work he did, he told the class that he hauled scrap metal all day long, which meant loading his truck with scrap metal, sometimes weighing up to 60 pounds, driving it across town and then unloading it.

"Believe me, I get all the exercise I need," he very confidently told the class. After a short walk down the hall and down one flight of stairs, my class of about six arrived at cardiac rehab. It was finally time for my scrap metal hauler to get on the treadmill and show us what good shape he was in! I oriented the patient as to how to use the treadmill and started him at a pretty conservative 2 mph. I then slowly increased the speed to about 2.5mph and told him to call me if he needed me.

I walked a few feet away to start two other gentlemen, both in their early 60's, on the treadmill. As I was trying to explain what these men needed to do to operate the treadmill, etc., I heard my scrap metal hauler complaining how I must be trying to kill him or something. I excused myself and went over to see what was going on with him. I ask him if he's messing around or if he is really tired.

"Yes, I'm dying here."

I slowed him down to about 2 mph. He seemed to be okay at that speed, and he began to catch his breath. As he recovered I explained that 2 mph for a man forty years old was considered pretty slow and introduced the idea that he apparently wasn't in as good of shape as he thought, and he agreed. I pointed out that the two gentlemen in their sixties were walking and talking quite comfortably at 3mph.

"So you don't think all that work I do at work is enough exercise?" he asked.

"What do you think," I asked him, "do you think if you were in good physical shape you would be having this much trouble walking on a treadmill at 2.5 mph?" He didn't respond right away, at least not verbally, but the expression on his face and the nodding of his head back and forth led me to believe that he wasn't in the shape he thought he was in and was frustrated about it. I explained that when he lifted scrap metal it was better than if he sat at a desk all day and did nothing but obviously was not enough exercise to keep him fit. I told him there were very few jobs physically active enough such that a regular exercise routine was not necessary. In other words almost everyone, whether they have diabetes or not, needs to follow a regular exercise routine regardless of what they do at work.

"How about if you work for the telephone company and you climb up and down telephone poles all day?" I have been asked that question before. That sounds pretty physical. But is it really? Consider this, what if you were given the task of following a telephone man on a typical workday? You were given a stopwatch and told to start it and let it run only when the phone man was actually climbing up or down the ladder. Don't let the stopwatch run when the telephone man is simply standing on the ladder working with his hands on the wires, just standing on a ladder is not exercise. No credit given. Don't let the watch run when the telephone man is driving from one work site to another. That surely doesn't count as exercise. No credit given. And by all means, don't let the stopwatch run while the telephone man is eating lunch. The stopwatch should only run when the telephone man is doing some physical activity.

Now, I have never followed a telephone man but I will try to be generous here. Let's say that through the course of a day's work the telephone man climbs up his ladder twenty five times. Let's say it is a very long ladder and he is a slow climber. It takes the man thirty seconds to climb up and another thirty seconds to climb down, round trip being about one minute. One minute per round trip at twenty- five trips makes for twenty- five minutes of exercise during the eight-hour workday. Put another way, one sixteenth of the workday is spent climbing up or down ladders. Granted this is far better then sitting behind a desk or computer all day but a far cry from "climbing ladders all day." In addition to the limited exercise this telephone man gets at work, he also needs a regularly performed exercise program.

5. Have you ever had a friend say something similar to this, "I spend about 2 1/2 hours at the gym just about every day? I'm always working out." Before you start getting overly impressed and envious of your friend's willpower, let me point out that "being at the gym" for 2 1/2 hours does not necessarily equate to exercising for 2 1/2 hours, in fact it rarely does. What you may not know is that this includes time in the locker room changing clothes, showering and talking. This does not include breaks at the water fountain or rest time between exercises that can be quite lengthy if you get involved in a conversation. Just as in the previous example about the telephone man, if you only count the amount of time the person is actually exercising it is frequently far less then what you may initially be led to believe.

In our exercise facility we ask that patients keep records of what they do, specifically how long they exercise per session, how many calories they burn, what their pre and post exercise blood sugars and blood pressures are, and that they log it in the computer. This way when a patient comes in to exercise eight weeks later and says, "By the way, I'm down from a size 14 to a size 10 since I started here," I can go to the computer, pull up her information and say that I'm not surprised when I see that she has exercised 16 out of the 20 days we are open per month and for an average of 65 minutes per visit.

In contrast, unfortunately, is when a patient complains of not seeing or feeling any improvement since starting to exercise 6 weeks ago. In this case I take the patient over to the computer to see exactly what he or she has been doing. Upon looking at the patient's data I see that in the last six weeks the patient has only exercised 8 times. The patient usually is in disbelief when seeing this and their comment is something like, "I can't believe this. This can't be right. I thought I had come a lot more than that. Is this why I haven't improved? I guess I need to start coming more often, huh?

Well of course my answer is yes, a lot more.

Keeping some sort of records of what you do can be very helpful when it comes to keeping you on track. The records can be as detailed or simple as you choose, but they are a good idea. A lot of times just writing down in a day planner or on your desk calendar how long you exercised that day is good enough.

Chapter 6
Food and Nutrition

You may have started to wonder when in this book about diabetes was I ever going to start talking about food and what you eat. After all this is a book about diabetes, a disease usually characterized by having too much sugar (glucose) in the blood. What diabetes book would be complete without a section on what you should and shouldn't eat?

A common request from patients is to find them a book or handout that will tell them what they can eat that won't cause their blood glucose levels to go too high.

Other patients didn't want a book like that; they wanted a book that would tell them exactly what to eat for breakfast, lunch and dinner. They wanted a preplanned meal plan or menu for each meal. "I just want something that's going to tell me what to eat. I don't want to have to figure it out at each meal," they say.

I have found that for most people with diabetes, their diabetes treatment centers around food. In fact, it has been my experience that the majority of questions patients have are regarding food.

I am hopeful that after reading this book, however, if your diabetes treatment is going to center around only one thing, it will be exercise. Ideally, you will give exercise, better nutrition and medications all the attention necessary to successfully control your diabetes. Maintaining good diabetes control should not center around one mode of treatment. That being said, without a doubt making good food choices is very important in achieving and maintaining good blood glucose control as well as reducing the blood lipid levels that so often become elevated with type 2 diabetes. This chapter will focus on the impact making good food choices can have on your diabetes.

The Significance of Better Nutrition: Improved nutrition is a necessity for the successful management of diabetes for a number of reasons, not only because of its effect on blood glucose levels, but also because of the significance it has on blood lipid control. Lipids are fats in the blood and are often elevated in people with diabetes. Increased blood pressure or hypertension is also frequently a problem. Both of these cardiovascular risk factors contribute to the higher levels of heart disease and stroke seen in patients with diabetes. There is also the impact better nutrition has on weight gain.

The impact of nutrition on type 2 diabetes will be fully explained in the sections to come.

Blood Glucose Levels

According to the American Diabetes Association blood glucose levels before meals should be between 90-130mg/dl. Peak blood glucose levels after meals should be less than 180mg/dl. (10) Blood glucose levels usually start to rise shortly after the first bite of food is taken and continue to rise for approximately an hour. At that time, the one-hour mark after starting the meal, the level of glucose in the blood should reach its maximal level. The time it takes for the blood glucose level to reach its maximal value after the meal may vary depending on several factors.

One factor is how much fat was eaten at the meal. The higher the quantity of fat consumed the longer it is going to take for the level of glucose to rise. Another contributing factor is how much insulin is circulating in the bloodstream at the time. Assuming the blood glucose reaches its peak at one hour after the meal, or thereabouts, it will then start going down. Ideally, it should gradually drop so that by the time it is time for the next meal the level of glucose in the blood is in the 90-130mg/dl. range. Keep in mind that if a snack is eaten between meals the blood glucose level just prior to the next meal should still be in the 90-130mg/dl. range. In most instances this means the snack can't be too big or contain too many carbohydrates or the desired pre meal blood sugar goals won't be achievable. An exception to this might be if the patient was eating the snack after exercising in order to prevent the blood glucose from going too low as a result of maybe too much exercise or to treat an already low blood glucose level. Achieving these blood glucose goals is what is likely to prevent or reduce the risks of developing the devastating micro vascular complications frequently caused by diabetes.

Eating Less

Conscientious eating or making good choices when it comes to eating has a major and immediate impact on blood glucose levels. Eating less carbohydrates or drinking fluids with less carbohydrates is probably the fastest and easiest way to improve blood glucose levels. How easy this method is of course depends on the difficulty a person has cutting back on their carbohydrates. Undoubtedly, this is easier for some people than it is for others. As an example, reducing the carbohydrate content of the breakfast meal by eating a slightly smaller bowl of cereal with half of a cut up banana instead of a whole one and 4 ounces of juice instead of 8 ounces could mean the difference between a blood sugar level two hours later of 220mg/dl. versus 160mg/dl., a big difference.

I mentioned earlier that the success people have with diabetes is mostly the cumulative result of how many sound choices they make regarding what they eat and their exercise versus how many unsound choices they make regarding the same. Obviously if patients are able to reduce the carbohydrate content of their breakfast as in the example and their blood glucose level two hours after was 160mg/dl. instead of 220mg/dl. that would be considered a sound choice. The more often patients do this, make sound choices and limit the amount of carbohydrates or sugar per meal, the better their blood glucose levels would be and their control of the diabetes in general.

Some patients I have seen have little problem with this and have a big advantage over those patients who constantly struggle with eating too many carbohydrates and sugar. For the patients who have such a difficult time limiting their intake of carbohydrates and sugar, the performance of aerobic exercise like walking, swimming or cycling becomes even more important. Depending on the situation, that is, barring any condition where a greater amount of exercise than is normally recommended might be harmful for these patients, more frequent or a longer duration of exercise might be helpful. Doing more exercise does not totally compensate for the increased carbohydrate intake, but it may help use up some of the excess carbohydrate above what is needed by the body for energy, etc., helping to maintain more desirable blood glucose levels after eating.

As an example, over the Thanksgiving weekend or Christmas holidays or even New Years, any holiday period when there is likely to be more eating than usual, I recommend patients increase the amount of exercise they do.

Making better food choices and reducing the carbohydrate intake, hereafter referred to as energy restriction, is also likely to contribute to weight loss. Eating less, even without weight loss, is associated with increased insulin sensitivity and significant improvements in blood glucose levels. In other words, eating less food should result in improvements in blood glucose levels before much if any weight is lost. (63,64)

Because of the increased insulin sensitivity that results from eating less, someone with newly diagnosed type 2 diabetes may be able to achieve and maintain good blood glucose control, at least for a while, just by eating less. The reason I say "for a while" instead of leading you to believe eating less will take care of you for a lifetime is because early on, soon after the onset of diabetes, there are still a good number of functioning beta cells remaining in the pancreas. It has been estimated that 50 percent of the beta cells are still functioning at the onset of diabetes. As time goes on it is likely that the number of functioning beta cells will continue to decrease. At some point in the future it is expected the number of functioning beta cells will be reduced to the point where they cannot produce the necessary insulin required to control blood glucose levels even when they are closely watching their carbohydrate intake.

This is when the doctor will usually say it is time to start taking medication. Sometimes the patient will be reluctant to start taking any medication and ask what other options are available. If the patient has not been exercising while restricting energy intake, which he should have, adding regular exercise now might provide enough assistance to avoid medication a bit longer. If exercise had been initiated much earlier, perhaps at the same time as energy restriction, the patient might not need medication, yet.

As I mentioned earlier, doctors will often tell a patient to try treating the diabetes with "diet and exercise" initially to see if that will work. The problem with that, as I indicated, is that the patient tends "not to hear" or disregard the exercise part of the doctor's recommendation and only focuses on the diet part. That's a big mistake, but I have already covered that, and you probably don't want me to go over that again.

One of the things I like to do with each class is have the following dialogue:

I start off by asking, "You folks with diabetes have too much sugar in your blood, don't you? You also have a more difficult time getting this sugar out of your blood and into your muscle, fat and liver cells than people without diabetes, don't you?"

They respond yes to both questions. I draw a picture on the board of a blood vessel with a lot of sugar in it, represented by a bunch "S's."

Now, in consideration of this, can you think of an immediate, easy way that you can improve the situation?

Sometimes I have to wait a moment for a response. Sometimes I have to give them the answer. Sometimes I just help them along a bit. "If you have a hard time getting sugar out of your blood and into your cells, what is one way you can help yourself ?" I ask.

"Put less sugar in your blood to begin with," answers someone, finally.

"That's right," I tell them. If you put less sugar in the blood by eating only one half of a baked potato instead of a whole one, and one roll or piece of bread instead of two or three, and a couple of bites of dessert instead of the whole thing, then you have reduced the amount of sugar entering the blood. The blood sugar level will not rise as high, first of all, and you don't have to worry about getting as much sugar out of the blood because you didn't put as much into the blood to begin with.

This dialogue discusses what I have stated previously, that if you have the ability to restrict your energy intake, you would be wise to do so. Blood glucose levels should improve if for no other reason because you have less sugar entering the blood and, therefore, less you have to worry about getting out. If you have trouble with this concept, then if I were you I would look at trying to increase the amount of physical activity you do assuming your health will allow you.

A reduction in carbohydrate intake, or energy restriction, as I have been referring to it lately, may lead to a reduction in body fat mass that should further reduce insulin resistance. This is particularly true if you maintain this energy restriction long term. Remember to keep in mind though that even with energy restriction, eating less, and the resulting improvements in blood glucose levels, weight reduction may not occur right away and rarely seems to be quick enough to suit the patient.

Weight loss is only of significance if it is a body fat reduction that causes the weight loss. Weight loss at the expense of lean body mass, muscle, is of no benefit and may actually worsen metabolic control. So actually, body fat reduction is a more correct term to use here instead of weight loss. A true reduction in body fat is of great benefit in reducing insulin resistance, and will be discussed in more detail later.

If weight loss does not occur with diet control alone, which many times it won't, and the patient would benefit from losing weight, which is almost always the case, to improve insulin resistance, lower blood glucose levels, blood pressure, etc., patients will usually need to include exercise as part of their treatment strategy.

Blood Lipid Control

Better nutrition is also vitally important in treating and or maintaining blood fat levels, also known as lipids. Hopefully, you remember from earlier that heart disease or stroke is usually what kills people with diabetes. The statistics tell us that two out of three people with diabetes die from heart disease. This is partly due to the damage that can occur to the vascular system as a result of having high levels of glucose and insulin in the blood, particularly in the first or second hour after a meal. Having too much insulin in the blood, known as hyperinsulinemia, is thought to cause inflammation of the blood vessels, which is proposed to contribute to heart disease.

Another big reason people with type 2 diabetes are at such high risk for developing heart disease is because so often they meet the criteria of having the metabolic syndrome, a clustering of various metabolic disorders. These typically include an increased waist circumference, insulin resistance, high blood pressure, elevated total cholesterol, LDL cholesterol and triglycerides, and low levels of the good cholesterol, the HDL's.

By definition, if you have three of the above disorders, you have the metabolic syndrome.

All of the disorders that comprise the metabolic syndrome are risk factors for heart disease. The more of these disorders a person has, the greater the likelihood of developing heart disease.

Unfortunately, many people with diabetes don't realize that they have to do more than just keep their blood glucose levels looking good and have a good HbA1C to stay healthy. That is what they need to do to reduce the risks of the micro vascular complications, retinopathy (eye disease), neuropathy (nerve disease), and nephropathy, (kidney disease), and somewhat reduce their risk of heart disease. Although the presence of the micro vascular diseases can certainly mess up the quality of life, these complications do not usually result in death. The macro vascular disease that results from not keeping the blood pressure and blood fats in check is what is largely responsible for the heart disease and two out of three people with diabetes dying from a heart attack or stroke. You don't want to become so focused on your blood sugar levels that you ignore your blood lipid profile and the fact that you may have some elevated values that need to be addressed by the doctor.

Consider this: Do you have any idea what your total cholesterol value was the last time it was checked? How about your low-density cholesterol, the really bad kind, do you know what it is? And how about your triglyceride level? And finally your HDL's, the good cholesterol, the kind of cholesterol that helps protect your heart, do you know those levels? I find many, many, times, in fact most of the time, when I pose these questions to participants in my class maybe two out of 10 patients know some of their values. Rarely does anyone know all of their values and most know none of them.

I then ask them if they know their cell phone number. Almost all do. I then ask them if they know their social security number. Again, almost all do. And finally I ask them if they know their checking account number. Most of them do. Quite a contrast between the answers concerning the numbers they use in day to day living and the numbers concerning their blood lipid control, the numbers indicating the risk of having a heart attack or stroke, the numbers that have to do with their health. Why do you suppose this is? Do you think it is odd that a group of people at high risk for heart disease, because of their diabetes, don't even know what their total cholesterol, LDL cholesterol or triglyceride levels are? Well, whether you find it odd or not, I find it to be very disconcerting.

Even the small percentage of patients who do know their values don't necessarily know if their values are good or not. Very few patients know what is considered the normal range for these blood fats. Even fewer know that the desirable range for these blood fats is lower for people with diabetes than what is considered normal for people without diabetes. Worded differently, many doctors want their patients with diabetes to achieve much lower blood fat levels than what is considered normal for the general population. This is because the risk of a person with diabetes developing heart disease is so much higher than in the general population; doctors hold their diabetes patients to a higher standard.

Did you know that the risk of a person with diabetes having their first heart attack is the same as for someone without diabetes who has already had one heart attack? If your doctor tells you that your labs are looking good, do you know which set of guidelines the doctor is following? Are they the guidelines for the general population or for someone with diabetes? Does your doctor distinguish between the two? Do you think you should know?

The accompanying table will tell you the generally recommended ranges for the blood fats discussed here as well as the range considered desirable for someone with diabetes.

It is of equal importance that you get your Hb A1C down below 7 percent and control your cardiovascular risk factors in order to significantly reduce your health risks and improve the odds of living the rest of your life complication free. That being said, improved nutrition can go a long way in helping control blood pressure and blood lipids.

So how can better nutrition improve blood lipid levels? Let's start off by discussing the role dietary fats play in your overall lipid profile.

Role of Dietary Fats

Fats play an enormous role in our daily diet. They make food taste good. If you were to take the fat out of our chocolate cake, our pizza, our ice cream and curly fries, we probably wouldn't eat as much of them, because they wouldn't taste as good. Without fat in our foods I believe we would all eat less, well at least the majority of us. I bet we would spend less time in restaurants, and fewer social occasions would center around food, in fact I bet there would be fewer social occasions.

Imagine having a Christmas party and serving all fat free foods. It might be the shortest party you ever hosted, but I'm sure it would get talked about. Fat is both good and bad. Good in that dietary fat makes foods taste good which in turn makes us want to eat. Just writing about it makes me want to jump off the couch and go see what we have to eat in the kitchen. Good because it insulates and cushions our bodies and good because it speeds up the transmission of nerve impulses. Bad because eating too much fat, more than our bodies need, will cause weight gain, making insulin resistance even worse than it might already be, high blood pressure, dyslipidemia (elevated lipid levels in the blood), arthritis, and sleep problems to name a few.

There are different kinds of dietary fat. Some of the fats, such as saturated fats and trans fats, can have more deleterious effects on blood lipid levels than others. Three other types of dietary fat known as monounsaturated, polyunsaturated and omega-3 polyunsaturated fat have a very positive effect on the lipid profile. The key here is to eat the right quantity of the right kinds of fats. This is the way it works. The three kinds of dietary fats most people are familiar with are saturated, polyunsaturated and monounsaturated. There is another fat called trans fat that is getting a lot of attention recently due to its reported association with heart disease.

There are 9 calories per gram of fat. It is the most dense, concentrated form of energy we eat. I say this because the same amount of carbohydrate and protein each have 4 calories per gram. This is true of all fats whether saturated, polyunsaturated or monounsaturated. Consuming an excess quantity of fat, any amount greater than your body needs, is going to contribute to weight gain and an increase in insulin resistance. Remember that any increase in body fat is going to increase insulin resistance.

Saturated fats and trans fats are known to raise blood cholesterol levels. (65)

Someone with type 2 diabetes already at high risk for heart disease, does not want to do anything that's going to raise the level of total cholesterol or LDL cholesterol in the blood. That would increase the risk for coronary heart disease even higher.

The intake of saturated fat is likely to raise levels of LDL cholesterol in addition to the already mentioned total cholesterol levels. Higher levels of LDL's are considered by many cardiologists to be of greater significance in causing coronary heart disease than the level of total cholesterol in the blood. It is advisable for everyone, whether they have diabetes or not, to reduce their consumption of saturated fats to reduce the risk of heart disease. For a large majority of people with type 2 diabetes it becomes even more important. The American Heart Association and the National Cholesterol Education Program recommend that less than 10 percent of the total daily calories come from saturated fats. (64,66) In fact some people may benefit by lowering their saturated fat intake to less than 7 percent of daily calories. (65)

Saturated fats are found in animal fats such as meat, butterfat, lard and bacon.

Other sources of saturated fats are dairy fat containing foods such as whole milk and cheese, coconut, palm and palm kernel oils and hydrogenated vegetable oils. (65)

Table 6 - American Diabetes Association Lipid Recommendations for people with type 2 diabetes (10)

LDL-Cholesterol	<100
HDL-Cholesterol*	>40
Triglyceride	<150

Units are in mg/dl.

*It is recommended that the HDL goal for women be increased by 10mg/dl.

Table 7 - American Association of Clinical Endocrinologists Lipid Recommendations for patients with type 2 diabetes and dyslipidemia (66,68)

	Target (mg/dL)	
Plasma lipid	Acceptable	Ideal
Total Cholesterol	<200	<170
LDL-C holesterol	<130	<100
HDL-Cholesterol	>35	>45
Non-HDL-Cholesterol*	<160	<130
Triglyceride	<200	<150

Units are in mg/dl.

*Total serum cholesterol minus HDL-Cholesterol

Table 8 - Reference range from typical laboratory results sheet (69)

LDL Cholesterol	<130
HDL Cholesterol	men >40 women >50
Triglycerides	<150

Units are in mg/dl.

Just as you might expect two different financial planners to have different opinions as to how much money should be set aside for retirement each month, two different physicians may have different opinions as to what LDL-cholesterol goals should be. Due to the higher risk of heart and circulatory disease in patients with diabetes, some doctors may follow the more strict guidelines established by The American Association of Clinical Endocrinologists, while still others follow the guidelines established by The American Diabetes Association. As an example, for LDL cholesterol, the fraction of cholesterol that is known as the "bad" one, the cholesterol most responsible for coronary artery disease, there is a 30 point difference between the value on a lab sheet and that which the American Association of Clinical Endocrinologists recommend.

More and more endocrinologists and other specialists are now recommending their patients strive to achieve levels of LDL cholesterol as low as 70mg/dl., or below, a sixty point difference, or approximately half the less than 130mg/dl. "normal" or reference range indicated on most laboratory printouts.

Polyunsaturated fat can help lower cholesterol levels. It would be considered one of the good fats. The recommendation is that <10 percent of your fat consumption be in the form of polyunsaturated fats. (66,70) Good sources of polyunsaturated fats are vegetable oils such as corn, safflower, soybean, sunflower and cottonseed oils. Walnuts are also a good source. (65)

If the polyunsaturated fats have a downside it would be their varied effects on HDL cholesterol levels.

Omega-3 polyunsaturated fat (fish oils) is helpful in lowering triglyceride levels in the blood. They also have anti platelet clotting properties. Fish from cold deep waters are good sources as well as fatty fish like salmon, herring, albacore tuna, mackerel and sardines. Some plant sources such as flax, walnuts and canola contain this kind of fat. (93,65)

Monounsaturated fat will lower total cholesterol levels but does not adversely affect the HDL level. Five to 15 percent of your total fat consumption should be in this form. (66,70) You can find monounsaturated fat in peanut, canola and olive oils, olives and nuts, but not walnuts. (65)

Sometimes when a person with diabetes tries to reduce the amount of sugar they consume they inadvertently end up eating greater amounts of fat. As I mentioned earlier, the two things that typically make food taste good are fat and sugar. When food manufacturers limit the quantity of sugar they put in a product, they may compensate by adding fat to ensure it will still have an appealing taste. Blood sugar levels may improve as a result of eating less sugar; however, if more fat is eaten as a consequence the bodyweight may stay the same or increase because of the increase in fat consumed.

Without a doubt eating less sugar will improve blood sugar levels even without a weight loss; however, if replacing the sugar content of a meal with fat results in a deterioration of blood lipid levels and an increase in bodyweight due to the greater caloric value of fat versus sugar, well, is it worth it? After all the lower blood sugar levels will reduce the risk of eye disease, nerve disease and kidney disease, but the higher fat intake will increase the risk of heart disease and having a stroke. I guess what it comes down to is asking if the extent of improvement seen in blood sugar levels is worth the increase in weight gain, increased insulin resistance, and worsening of blood lipid levels.

Obviously a much better situation is if the sugar intake is reduced without a compensatory increase in fat intake. In this case not only are blood sugar levels improved but usually with no weight gain and frequently with a weight loss that should decrease insulin resistance. With no increase in the consumption of dietary fat there is no reason for the blood lipid level to worsen.

The only possible negative consequence to eating less fat, that I can think of, regardless of the type, is that the level of HDL cholesterol in the blood may drop.

Role of Protein

Protein is used extensively in the human body, not just for building muscle, but also for most if not all life sustaining processes. In this country, protein constitutes approximately 15-20 percent of the average adult's energy intake. This represents about twice the recommended daily allowance or RDA for protein. There is some evidence to show that consuming this quantity of protein is related to the development of nephropathy. (71)

Most adults are able to meet their protein needs by consuming 1gram of protein per kilogram of bodyweight. As for most children, adolescents, and athletes, they can meet their protein needs with 1.2 grams per kilogram of bodyweight. (65)

As far as the role protein plays in diabetes, it depends largely on whether the patient's blood sugar is in control or not. If blood sugar levels are in good control the consumption of protein has little effect on blood sugar levels. Conversely, if the level of insulin in the blood is inadequate and blood sugar levels are elevated, then the consumption of protein may result in a further deterioration of blood sugar control. For people with diabetes who still have the ability to manufacture insulin in the beta cells of the pancreas, protein consumption can stimulate the production and release of insulin just as well as sugar consumption. (72,73)

It has been suggested that by consuming protein at the same time as carbohydrate the carbohydrate will cause a slower and less severe rise in blood sugar levels as compared to eating the carbohydrate by itself. Contrary to this belief, the peak insulin response is similar whether carbohydrate is consumed alone or with protein. (72)

People that tend to have their blood sugar levels drop too low in the middle of the night while sleeping are often told to take a small snack before bed. This is usually a snack containing a small amount of carbohydrate. It has been suggested that by adding protein to the carbohydrate snack the carbohydrate is more likely to sustain the blood sugar during the night. This may or may not help, but there seems to be no hard and fast rule regarding this.

Protein provides 4 calories of energy per gram. This is slightly less than half the energy provided when 1 gram of fat is metabolized. As I have already mentioned, fat is energy and calorie rich, whereas protein and carbohydrates are not. As long as protein intake is not unusually low or high and falls near the recommendations mentioned above, there is probably no reason to make any adjustments as far as protein is concerned.

Role of Carbohydrates

Carbohydrate is not a bad word. You shouldn't cringe or make ugly disparaging faces or remarks when you hear the word 'carbohydrates.' Nor should you cringe or make faces when you hear the word 'sugar,' which is also not a bad word. In fact, carbohydrates, of which sugar is one, are quite necessary and we could not get by without them.

They sure have gotten a bad reputation though. You give a child too many carbohydrates and they are blamed for "kids bouncing off the walls" and being hyper. Carbohydrates, or too many carbohydrates, are blamed for weight gain. Carbohydrates, namely sugar, are blamed for tooth decay. When is someone going to come to the aid of carbohydrates? To date the only people I have ever known that have spoken favorably of carbohydrates are athletes, particularly long distance or endurance athletes. Experienced endurance athletes are all too familiar with the pitfalls of eating too little carbohydrates and the benefits of eating meals high in carbohydrates, also known as carbohydrate loading.

Carbohydrates are the body's fuel of choice. They are readily available and can be metabolized quickly, providing an almost immediate source of energy. It takes twice as much carbohydrate to provide the same amount of energy as half the amount of fat, but it is a lot easier and quicker to metabolize than fat, making it the fuel of choice.

Carbohydrates are used almost exclusively for any vigorous activity-such as running, jogging and even very brisk walking-that requires a constant supply of readily available energy. When the intensity of the exercise drops and the rate at which energy needs to be supplied slows a bit, there is a shift towards using greater amounts of fat for energy.

Endurance athletes run out of gas prematurely when competing in long endurance events if sufficient carbohydrates are not eaten prior to the competition. Athletes refer to running out of carbohydrates before the end of a race as "hitting the wall," a very real, unpleasant feeling, that comes upon the athlete when their carbohydrate fuel sources are low and the body shifts from mainly carbohydrate metabolism to predominately fat metabolism. Prior to competitive events endurance athletes typically "load up" on carbohydrates 24-48 hours before the event to help ensure they will have enough fuel to complete the event.

One of the benefits of doing all of the training these athletes do is that they become able to store more carbohydrate in their muscles and liver that can be used when called upon. It's like these athletes have bigger fuel tanks than everyone else.

In addition to the practice of carbohydrate loading before a race, many endurance athletes maintain a high carbohydrate intake pretty much all the time. The idea behind this is that some athletes believe they train so long and hard that they need to replenish their muscle and liver stores with greater than normal amounts of carbohydrate on a daily basis.

So here we have an example of where eating larger than normal quantities of carbohydrate can be beneficial, for certain groups of people that is. For most people this would not be the case and for someone with diabetes it would definitely not be the case.

Let's look at drinking alcohol for a minute. Various studies have suggested that drinking small amounts of alcohol may be helpful in treating certain medical conditions, but we also know that drinking alcohol in excess can have disastrous consequences. Now, whether alcohol is regarded as good or bad depends largely on how much is consumed and the effect it has on the person consuming it. I will have more to say about alcohol later.

Carbohydrates can be viewed much the same way. Eating a diet high in carbohydrates can be very beneficial for endurance athletes, particularly before a long race, but for someone with diabetes a diet high in carbohydrates can be quite harmful.

Carbohydrates are not bad when the right amount is consumed. If people without diabetes maintain a good bodyweight and get plenty of exercise, there is nothing wrong with eating a moderate quantity of carbohydrate, and it should not affect them adversely. (Keep in mind I am speaking from a diabetes perspective, I cannot comment on carbohydrate's effect on teeth.) If over a period of time, such as the Christmas and New Years holidays or a vacation, as an example, some of these people overdo it with the carbohydrates a bit, as long as they don't put any weight on and continue to exercise, it shouldn't be a problem. If, however, a time came when these people quit exercising, put some weight on and still ate a moderate quantity of carbohydrates, that wouldn't be so good. Carbohydrates themselves are still not bad, but eating a moderate to large portion of them under those circumstances would be a bad idea.

Have you ever been surprised to see a retired professional athlete, such as a football or baseball player, look a lot bigger, fatter, than during his playing years? What often happens is that after the athlete retires the amount of exercise they get goes way down but the amount of food they eat does not. The result is an abundance of unspent calories leading to an over weight, out of condition candidate for diabetes. I would bet money the athlete is already a member in good standing of the metabolic syndrome club. How could diabetes not be far behind?

Let's say a person with diabetes really, really likes to eat carbohydrates, more than they should. If this person is someone that likes to exercise and is willing to do more exercise to compensate for the increase in carbohydrates they may be able to, in a sense, get away with it, however, if an increase in the person's exercise does not happen, then the quantity of carbohydrates eaten needs to be watched more carefully.

Limiting carbohydrate intake is the way a lot of people with diabetes would like to control their illness. "I'll just eat less carbohydrates," they will say. This may seem to work early on, however, considering that diabetes is a progressive illness it is realistic to expect that frequent further reductions in carbohydrate intake will be necessary in order to maintain good blood sugar control. Eventually though, even eating a very small amount of carbohydrate may send the blood sugar levels too high as more and more beta cells continue to become dysfunctional. Eating fewer carbohydrates is not enough, not in the long run.

More on Carbohydrates

Before getting into a more in depth discussion about carbohydrates, it would be a good idea to take some time to introduce and define the terms I will be using.

A carbohydrate is a chemical compound that contains carbon, hydrogen and oxygen.

You might say to that, "I never took chemistry, that doesn't mean anything to me."

Well, that's okay, I understand. But I will tell you that it is because of the unique composition of carbohydrates, what they are made of, and how they are put together, that makes them easy to metabolize and good sources of energy.

There are three types of carbohydrates. They are known as sugars, starch and fiber. (74)

Saccharide is Latin for sugar.

Sugars are referred to as monosaccharides and disaccharides. Polysaccharides are starches and fiber.

A monosaccharide is the simplest form of sugar. It consists of one sugar.

Monosaccharides are the building blocks of disaccharides like sucrose, table sugar.

A disaccharide is a sugar composed of two monosaccharides.

Now, just so you know, I am explaining this for those of you who have a thirst for this kind of information. For those of you not that interested in knowing exactly what a monosaccharide or polysaccharide are, that's perfectly okay. You can still take good care of your diabetes without knowing this. Don't sweat it.

An oligosaccharide contains anywhere from three to ten sugars. We are not going to discuss oligosaccharides beyond giving the definition, as there is no need.

A polysaccharide contains many, many sugars. (75)

Two good examples of monosaccharides are glucose and fructose. As for disaccharides, sucrose and lactose are good examples. (76) Galactose comes from lactose which is milk sugar. I'm sure you have heard the term "lactose intolerant." If someone is lactose intolerant they have lost the ability to properly digest the sugar lactose.

People have often believed that eating foods with white, table sugar in them, or putting table sugar in coffee or tea was terribly harmful for someone with diabetes. It's not.

You may be surprised to learn that some sugars, namely, fructose, lactose and sucrose may have less of an impact on raising blood sugar levels than starches and glucose. (76) Yes, that large baked potato, a starch, with all those "complex carbohydrates," an outdated and no longer recognized term, is likely to wreak more havoc with blood sugar levels than the sugar you sweetened your iced tea with and put on your morning bowl of cereal.

The reason for this is that when metabolized some of these sugars (fructose, lactose and sucrose) are converted to glycogen and stored in the liver or converted to triglycerides. As a result only small amounts of these sugars are converted to glucose and overall blood sugar, (glucose) levels may not rise as much as you might expect.

Starches are polysaccharides as is dietary fiber. (76)

If you remember from above, polysaccharides contain many, many sugars. Perhaps this is the reason starches are likely to have a greater impact on raising blood sugar levels than the sugars, fructose, lactose and sucrose. Good sources of starches are cereal, grains, starchy vegetables (potatoes, winter squash, peas and corn), and legumes (peas, beans and lentils). (65)

The ability of a starch to be digested quickly and to what extent it is digested depends largely on three factors: the structure of the starch, how it comes packaged in the plant source and how it is processed or cooked. The message here is that starches, (polysaccharides), have more of a tendency to raise blood sugar levels than sucrose, (cane sugar), fructose, (sugar coming from fruit and some vegetables), and lactose, (milk sugar).

Polysaccharide carbohydrate components of plants that are non-starch and non-digestible are known as dietary or food fiber. This may be sometimes referred to as cellulose. The ingestion of dietary fiber is thought to have little impact on blood glucose levels, however, when I discuss carbohydrate counting in the next section you will see where fiber intake is considered into the counting of carbohydrates. Whether or not fiber has an effect on blood glucose levels, there is reason to believe that the ingestion of fiber may help lower LDL cholesterol levels. (65) A person with diabetes should follow the same guidelines for fiber intake as the general population. (74,77) These guidelines call for the inclusion of a variety of fiber containing foods including whole grains, fruits and vegetables. And keep in mind that the vitamins, minerals and fiber they contain play a significant role in maintaining good health. (78)

Blood pressure is oftentimes elevated in patients who have diabetes. It is recommended that the blood pressure not exceed 130/80mm/Hg for patients with diabetes. Following good nutrition practices, and particularly, watching the sodium and caffeine consumption can have a significant impact on blood pressure levels. It has been reported that people with diabetes are more salt sensitive than people without diabetes, reinforcing the need to keep closer watch on salt consumption. (79)

It is recommended that sodium consumption be limited to less than 2400mg/day. (78,80) The Dietary Approaches to Stop Hypertension (DASH) sodium study provides information that encourages a reduced sodium intake. (81) Just one teaspoon of salt, which is 5 grams, contains 2300 mg of sodium, approximately the maximum that is recommended for daily consumption. (65) A low sodium food as defined by the FDA is having less than 140 mg or less of sodium per serving. Reading food labels is a good way to get an idea of how much sodium is in the foods you are eating. The sodium listed is per serving. For some people, particularly those who are described as salt sensitive, restricting salt intake may be enough to maintain good blood pressure control. In others, medications may be necessary to arrive at goal.

Another consideration is the impact nutrition has on weight gain and weight loss. One of the worst things a person with diabetes can do is gain weight, that is, if the weight is in the form of fat. Conversely, as has already been discussed, losing weight, if the weight lost is fat mass, is just about the best thing someone with diabetes can do, particularly if accompanied by exercise.

Eating less sugar, over time, may lead to weight loss. If weight loss does occur, then eating less sugar has contributed to decreasing insulin resistance, in other words, knocking some of the rust off of the rusty hinges. This means that the doors to the muscle, fat and liver cells will become easier to open, thus requiring less insulin. Anytime something can be done to make life easier for the beta cells, so they don't have to work so hard, that is a very good thing.

If weight loss does not occur with a reduced sugar intake, which it may not, particularly if other non sugar but higher in fat foods are substituted for foods containing sugar, then insulin resistance will not likely improve. Remember, anytime fat mass in the body can be reduced, even as little as ten pounds, there is a corresponding improvement (decrease) in insulin resistance. It of course would still be a great idea to consume less sugar, even if weight loss didn't occur, because of the reduced levels of sugar in the blood and improved HbA1C score.

Body Fat

As body fat mass is reduced, blood sugar levels improve as well as insulin resistance. In fact caloric restriction in general decreases insulin resistance. (82) In the United Kingdom Prospective Diabetes Study, the HbA1C improved by 2 percent in the first 3 months with intensive diet. That is really good. This was the most significant drop in HbA1C seen throughout the study. During the initial three-month period, not only did the HbA1C drop nicely but the same participants saw a 5 percent weight loss. (83) The authors of the study concluded, however, that the initial improvement in blood sugar levels was more related to the lack of food consumed than to weight loss. The reduction in bodyweight was thought to be a secondary response. (83) Furthermore, the study showed that fasting blood sugars went back up in patients who did not continue to follow a restricted caloric intake. This occurred even when the weight loss was maintained. (83)

When improved diet alone results in weight loss, it is conceivable that blood sugar control may improve a great deal and that this improvement may last for an extended period of time without additional short-term intervention. It is the opinion of many experts that losing weight in the form of body fat is likely to be the single most important factor in reducing insulin resistance, thereby improving the diabetes.

Although losing bodyweight by caloric restriction alone is possible and happens everyday, research as well as anecdotal reports, indicates that within a one to two year period after weight loss a majority of the weight that was lost returns and sometimes more. Better results are seen when a reduced caloric intake is combined with a program of regular exercise.

Unfortunately, in many instances once blood glucose levels have improved and weight loss has occurred, many people reduce the exercise or discontinue it altogether.

Even though blood sugar levels may improve significantly for some patients with only caloric restriction, at least for a while, I would wholeheartedly recommend initiating exercise as soon after receiving the diagnosis as possible. Improvements in blood sugar levels associated with caloric restriction and carbohydrate reduction alone are likely to be magnified when exercise is initiated at the same time.

The combination of regular exercise and initiating what I call a "diabetes conscious meal plan," soon after the diagnosis of diabetes should lead to good metabolic control, which of course is the ultimate goal. Although it is very important to lose excess body fat for an assortment of health reasons, including reducing insulin resistance, the main emphasis should be on achieving and maintaining good metabolic control. (65) Therefore, it is possible to achieve good blood glucose control when carrying excess body fat, but more difficult due to the higher degree of insulin resistance that comes with the extra fat. If blood glucose goals can be achieved in spite of the excess body fat, that's great, but every effort should still be made to lose the fat because of its deleterious influence on insulin resistance, blood pressure and remaining cardiovascular risk factors.

Carbohydrate Counting

Perhaps you have heard of carbohydrate counting before, maybe not. A lot of people with diabetes use carbohydrate counting and then there are a lot of people who don't "count their carbs" as it is often referred to. What I am getting at here is that counting your carbohydrates is something that can be very useful in helping manage blood glucose levels, but it is not absolutely necessary for everyone to do it. You may be able to very successfully manage blood sugars without actually counting the carbs. I believe that most people with diabetes actually do some form of carbohydrate counting whether they realize it or not. I think a lot of people have some kind of idea of how many or how much in the way of carbohydrates they consume on a daily basis. In the next several pages I will explain carbohydrate counting and how it can be used to better control blood glucose levels.

This is how you do it. When counting carbohydrates, the focus is on the total quantity of carbohydrate consumed, not where the carbohydrate came from. Eating a variety of foods from all of the major food groups and striving to achieve healthy eating patterns is the ultimate goal, while still keeping an eye on the total carbohydrates consumed.

To count carbohydrates you first start by dividing foods into 3 food groups: carbohydrate, meat and meat substitutes, and fat. (65) One serving of carbohydrate contains 15 grams of carbohydrate. Foods that contain carbohydrate are starches, fruits, milk and desserts. Starchy vegetables like potatoes, corn, peas, and winter squash are also considered carbohydrate servings. (65) Vegetables are sources of carbohydrate but contain only small amounts. Green and leafy vegetables or a plate of cooked vegetables only count if a large quantity is consumed.

Meats contain no carbohydrate. An average serving of meat, fish, or poultry is three ounces or about the size of a deck of cards. (65) If your meal consisted of 4 hot dogs, with no buns of course, then your carbohydrate count would be zero. A nice juicy, steak, but no baked or mashed potatoes, still no carbohydrates. You might quickly jump to the conclusion, "Hey, I love meat, I'll just focus on eating more meats and keep my carbohydrates down. I can do that." Not so fast. Granted, there are no carbohydrates in meat, but there can be plenty of fat, depending on the cut of meat, of course. As discussed earlier, you want to keep the fat content down. A diet of predominantly meat would make it very difficult to keep the saturated fat content down.

The other problem with this example is that you don't want a meal without any carbohydrates. There should be carbohydrates in every meal. Avoiding carbohydrates to the extent that you are not consuming any at any given meal is likely to lead to problems with hypoglycemia.

As for meat substitutes, an average serving of a meat substitute is 1 ounce of cheese, ½ cup cottage cheese, 1 egg, or 1 Tbsp peanut butter. Again, there are no carbohydrates here but there is fat.

Then there is fat. Fat contains no carbohydrate and will not contribute to the carbohydrate count either. Each serving of fat does contain approximately five grams of fat, though, and therefore, if more is consumed than the body needs will contribute to weight gain. Examples of a fat serving are 1 tsp of butter, margarine, mayonnaise, or regular salad dressing; and 2 Tbsp of reduced fat salad dressing, cream cheese, or sour cream. (65)

When people first start to count carbohydrates there needs to be a point at which to start from. I think people refer to this as the jumping off point. For the average type 2 adult it is common for a female to start with three to four carbohydrate servings per meal (45 to 60 grams) and a male to start with four to five carbohydrate servings per meal (60 to 75 grams). One snack, either mid morning, afternoon, or evening of one to two carbohydrate servings (15 to 30 grams), is acceptable to start with.

Just as important as counting carbohydrates is testing the blood glucose levels to see if the overall blood glucose control is where it should be. This usually will require testing blood sugar levels three to four times per day, initially, and then backing off to maybe two to three times per day later on. If blood glucose levels are too high following a meal, then it may mean the quantity of carbohydrates for that meal needs to be reduced a bit. Remember that the American Diabetes Association recommends peak postprandial (after meal) blood glucose levels not exceed 180mg/dl. (10)

For some men four to five carbohydrates per meal may simply be too many due to their lack of physical activity and body size. In this case reducing the carbohydrates to four in the morning (60 grams) and evening (60 grams), with three at lunch (45 grams) might bring the blood glucose levels in line very well.

Keep in mind that the foremost goal of eating is to provide the body with adequate vitamins, minerals and energy for proper maintenance, growth and development. Healthy foods providing nourishment to the body should never be sacrificed or minimized to allow for a better blood glucose value after eating. Good nutrition comes first; then if blood sugar levels are not what they need to be after meals, consideration should be given to increasing physical activity during the day or talking to the doctor about adjusting medications. When there is less variation in the amount of carbohydrate eaten at each meal, there should be less variation in postprandial blood sugar levels. In some cases, when there is variation in the carbohydrate content of a meal and when the patient is insulin requiring, the healthcare team instructs the patient regarding how to make adjustments in the insulin dosage to accommodate changes in carbohydrate. This should only be attempted with the consent of the patient's doctor and only when the patient is insulin requiring.

Some patients routinely eat too many carbohydrates and then, in order to maintain good blood glucose control, take extra insulin to help get the extra sugar out of the blood and into the cells. Doing this once in a while should not be a significant problem; however, when done frequently it is a bad idea and likely to cause weight gain. This would be a case of misusing insulin. The weight gain is caused when the extra insulin, above what is usually injected, picks up the sugar from the blood and helps it enter the muscle, fat and liver cells. Once in the muscle or fat cells, if not used, the sugar is stored as fat.

Reading Food Labels

When reading the label on any food product pay particular attention to the number of servings because the numbers you see listed are based on one serving, not the whole box or whole package. Near the top of the label it will say serving size and servings per container. You need to look for total carbohydrate next. Total carbohydrate includes all of the starches, sugars and fiber. Don't pay any attention to the part that states the grams of sugar. That is included in the total carbohydrate. As an example, the serving size may be 8 ounces, servings per container 4, total carbohydrates 38, and calories 152. Now, if you drink the contents of the whole container, you have consumed 32 ounces, total carbohydrate 152 grams and calories 608. Got the idea?

One more thing, when you find the quantity of fiber per serving, if the amount is 5 grams or more, this amount can be subtracted from the total carbohydrate before converting the total grams of carbohydrate into servings.

Determining the Insulin-to-Carbohydrate Ratio

Insulin-to-carbohydrate ratios are only used for patients who are injecting insulin. The insulin-to-carbohydrate ratio can be defined as the amount of insulin required to adequately control blood sugars when a given amount of carbohydrate is consumed.

To determine the ratio you first need to make sure the blood sugars are under reasonably good control, with average blood sugar levels less than 200 mg/dl. You then need to eat a consistent number of carbohydrates for at least three days and figure out how much mealtime quick acting insulin you need to keep your blood sugar level where you want it.

You then take the total grams of carbohydrate eaten at a meal and divide that number by number of units of insulin taken just before the meal. The resulting number will be your insulin-to-carbohydrate ratio.

As an example, let's say you consume 75 grams of carbohydrate and take 5 units of quick acting insulin. Divide 5 into 75 and you come up with 15. This means that 1 unit of insulin is needed for every 15 grams of carbohydrate consumed. Patients more sensitive to the effects of insulin may have carbohydrate-to-insulin ratios of 1:20, 1:25, etc. Patients who are more insulin resistant may have ratios of 1:10, 1:5, etc. As the course of diabetes progresses a patient may find that the insulin-to-carbohydrate ratio changes. The direction and magnitude of the change to a large extent is the result of what the patient is doing to take care of their diabetes. As an example, if a patient exercises regularly, eats sensibly and loses some weight the ratio may go from 1:15 to 1:20. Conversely, if little is done to improve insulin resistance and because type 2 diabetes is a progressive illness, the insulin-to-carbohydrate ratio may go from 1:15 to 1:10 or worse.

Vitamins and Minerals

When reviewing a list of medications a patient is taking it is a very common occurrence to see that in addition to the prescribed medications there are a number of vitamins, herbs or minerals the patient is taking. When I ask why these are being taken, the patient will tell me they read or saw online that these supplements were good for people with diabetes. There indeed have been many, many claims about various supplements, be it vitamins, minerals or herbs, that will in some way help control or cure diabetes. Most if not all of these supplements have been investigated, or are currently being investigated and so far appear to be generally safe, although to date there is no conclusive scientific evidence to support their use. (84) There are several supplements that have been studied that do warrant further investigation. (84) Until such time as there is sufficient scientific evidence to show the benefit and safety of these supplements and herbs their use cannot be endorsed.

There is a potential danger in taking commercially prepared herbs and vitamins as they are not regulated by the Food and Drug Administration and their content may vary. Additionally, some vitamins and minerals can cause serious problems when taken in large doses, not to mention that dangerous interactions may occur when taking certain prescription drugs. These are just some of the reasons it would be wise to discuss the use of any non-prescribed herb, vitamin or supplement with your doctor and pharmacist.

Alcohol

People with diabetes need to be even more cautious when consuming alcohol than the general population. An increased risk of hypoglycemia is occurs when people with diabetes drink alcohol of any kind, be it beer, wine, liquor, etc. This is because alcohol is absorbed from the stomach and small intestine and metabolized in the liver as a fat. Alcohol is not a fat, but because of its chemical structure it is treated as one by the liver and when metabolized does not lead to an increase in the blood sugar level as carbohydrates would. There is nothing really problematic with that except that because alcohol has a toxic effect on the liver it prevents the liver from doing one of its most important jobs, which is to release sugar into the blood when levels of sugar in the blood start dropping too low, thus resulting in hypoglycemia.

Regardless of the cause, when blood glucose levels start to drop, the liver is temporarily prevented from releasing sugar into the blood if alcohol has recently been consumed or is being consumed. Therefore, the "safety net," as I prefer to think of the liver, cannot step in and prevent the blood glucose level from dropping even further, much less raise it to normal levels. In effect the alcohol temporarily paralyzes this important function of the liver.

If a diabetes patient is planning on having an alcoholic drink or two without having something to eat at the same time, she should check to see that the blood sugar level is in a good safe range and high enough to prevent a hypoglycemic problem that might occur if it did start to drop a bit. The safest thing to do of course is to always eat some food along with the alcoholic beverage. Did you notice that I said beverage? That wasn't by accident, particularly if you are a female. Women should have no more than one alcoholic drink per day and men no more than two. (46) A frequent question is what constitutes one drink? That's a great question. An alcoholic drink can be defined as 12 ounces of beer, 5 ounces of wine, or 1½ ounces of hard liquor (distilled spirits).

Here is another topic that frequently arises: Let's say you ate some food in the afternoon to go along with your drink as suggested. Let's say it was 15 or 30 grams of carbohydrate. Should you subtract that amount of carbohydrate from your next meal? The answer is definitely no. No food should be subtracted from the next meal to compensate for the food taken with the alcohol. (74)

There is epidemiological evidence suggesting that for non-diabetic adults having one to two drinks per day reduces the risk for type 2 diabetes, coronary artery disease, and stroke. (85,86,87) Other studies have shown that consuming this amount of alcohol can increase insulin sensitivity. (116,117)

As for people with type 2 diabetes, what effect does light to moderate drinking have on them? Studies have reported a decreased risk of coronary artery disease for both men and women. (90,91,92) This may be due to an increase in HDL cholesterol levels. (89) Anyone drinking alcohol and looking for these kinds of benefits must be careful not to cross the line between moderate and excessive drinking as excessive drinking can elevate blood pressure as well as worsen blood glucose control. This, of course, is in addition to the other negative consequences associated with excessive drinking.

Chapter 7
Medications

There is a common misconception that the more pills or medications you take for your diabetes the worse off you are. This is not necessarily the case. There is the misconception that if you take insulin injections to treat your diabetes, you are even worse off than those that do not take insulin. Again, not necessarily true. I have seen patients who were told or believe that they have "a little diabetes" or "a touch of sugar" who don't take any diabetes medication; however, they are already starting to experience at least one or more of the complications that results from poorly controlled diabetes. Sound puzzling? Let me explain.

When first diagnosed, many patients do not require medication to control their diabetes, particularly those who start exercising and making better choices as to what they eat. As for other patients, perhaps those who have had diabetes for a while without even knowing it, they may need medication from the start, and in some cases a lot of it, maybe even insulin.

If diagnosed immediately after developing diabetes, it is likely a good many patients could control their diabetes with better nutrition and exercise. As time goes on, however, the general feeling amongst most educators and physicians is that medication will become necessary at some point as more and more of the beta cells in the pancreas cease to function. Many times patients have had type 2 diabetes for quite sometime when it is eventually diagnosed, sometimes years, and just didn't know it. By the time these patients finally learn they have diabetes, too many of the beta cells have already ceased to function, and they are way past the stage when exercise and better nutrition alone will control their diabetes. These patients missed that stage altogether and most of them will move right into oral therapy and possibly even insulin therapy if the majority of beta cells have stopped functioning.

The thing about it is this: Diabetes is considered by most physicians and educators to be a progressive illness. As time goes by more and more beta cells will become exhausted from over work and stop working resulting in the need for increasing medication. When a sufficient number of beta cells have quit working, even maximal doses of the oral medications will not be able to control blood glucose levels. This is the time when the physician would typically recommend either adding insulin to the treatment regimen or switching to insulin altogether. In general, it is safe to say that if someone has type 2 diabetes for a long enough period of time, there is a good chance that eventually, someday, they will need supplemental insulin. It is important to point out here that the need to switch to insulin from pills does not necessarily represent any kind of poor management or failure on the part of the patient.

Glucose Toxicity

Until recently, when a physician started a patient on insulin, it was usually, but not always, because even with oral diabetes medications, the beta cells were no longer capable of making adequate insulin to maintain good blood glucose control. Physicians sometimes prescribe insulin for a patient at the time of diagnosis if the physician has found the patient's blood glucose is exceptionally high, say, over 300mg/dl.

When circulating levels of sugar in the blood are this high, they can have a toxic effect on the beta cells and further restrict their ability to make insulin. This is a condition commonly referred to as glucose toxicity. In this situation, the short-term use of insulin injections is used to supplement the endogenous insulin the beta cells are already producing. The goal here is to quickly get the blood glucose level down to more reasonable levels. Once achieved, the beta cells are no longer surrounded with this sugar rich blood, and the beta cells should be able to work better. With the glucose toxicity resolved, frequently, the oral medications are sufficient to maintain blood glucose levels, that is, assuming the patient is using relatively good judgment with food selection and exercise.

There is now evidence to show that intensive insulin therapy in patients with newly diagnosed type 2 diabetes can significantly improve beta cell function and facilitate further long-term blood glucose control. (93) In light of this information more physicians are adding insulin or switching to insulin from oral medications much earlier in the treatment regimen.

Until recently, in most cases, physicians did not suggest a patient begin using insulin until it was felt the oral medications or a combination of oral medications were no longer effective in controlling blood glucose levels. Healthcare professionals have sometimes threatened patients with insulin, indicating that if they did not get their blood glucose levels under control within a specified period of time that they would be switched to insulin injections. This is not the best approach to take when starting someone off on the road to taking insulin! It is likely that a great many patients with type 2 diabetes are likely to require insulin injections at some point in their lifetime to control their diabetes due to the progressive nature of the disease. If the patient has been told on various occasions, or even one time, that if they didn't do this or that to get the blood glucose levels under control, they will be started on insulin therapy, then whenever insulin therapy is initiated, now or later, patients are likely to feel they have failed and that it is their fault they must now take insulin.

"Being where you need to be is sometimes more important than how you got there."

With diabetes it's not what medications you take and how much that matters; it's how well you control your blood glucose levels. Consider this: let's say you have two patients, Bob and Jim. Bob has an HbA1C of 6.5 percent and takes 5mg. of glipizide, 15 mg. of rosiglitazone and 1000mg. of metformin. Jim has a HbA1C of 8.5 percent but takes only 15 mg. of rosiglitazone. Which patient is worse off? Bob, who takes a lot of diabetes medicine but has a low HbA1C of 6.5 percent, or Jim who takes only a little diabetes medicine and has a HbA1C of 8.5 percent? Jim is in worse shape because he has a higher HbA1C. It's the HbA1C that indicates how well or how poorly a person is managing their diabetes, not how many medications it takes to get there. Certainly it's nicer to be able to maintain good blood glucose control with less medication; it's less trouble and less expensive but not always possible. Instead of struggling with it and being unsuccessful at trying to keep the blood glucose levels in good control with little or no medication, it would be much wiser to take more medication and get the blood glucose levels in the desired range.

Imagine this scenario: Let's say there were two major forest fires burning out of control. One was in your county while the other was in the next county. You were the fire chief in one county and your best friend was the fire chief in the neighboring county. Significant damage was being done and the pressure was on to get the fire under control and, eventually, extinguished. Knowing your job was on the line you made use of every technique you knew to contain the fire. You lined up a hundred men on the south side of the fire and sprayed gallons of water on the blaze. Another fifty men dug trenches on the east side of the fire. Twenty men burned controlled backfires to the west of the fire. From above helicopters dropped fire retardants on the fire.

Your friend in the next county chose to line up two hundred firefighters on the south side of the fire and spray water on the fire twenty four hours a day. Which fire was brought under control the quickest and why? Your fire was because you fought the fire more aggressively using every firefighting technique you knew.

The important thing here is to get the fire under control as quickly as possible. You did, using every technique or method you could. You could say the same is true for diabetes. You want to get the blood glucose levels down to desirable ranges as quickly as possible to reduce the risks of long term complications. By treating the diabetes with two or three different types of medication you can effectively address all three of the problems contributing to elevated blood glucose levels and usually accomplish the goal of a lower HbA1C much sooner. Although all diabetes medications work to improve blood glucose control, they do not all work the same way, and in fact, there are approximately a half dozen different kinds, or classes, of diabetes medications. Most of these medications have been developed within the last ten years and have had a major impact in the treatment of diabetes.

Major Classes of Diabetes Medications

Sulfonylureas, Meglitinides, Phenylalanine derivatives, Biguanides, Thiazolidinediones, Alpha-glucosidase Inhibitors, Incretins and Gliptins. Do you think you can remember these? How about long term, for more than a day or two? Maybe not, and it's not like you really need to either. Your doctor or pharmacist or a diabetes educator will frequently use these names when discussing medications with other professionals; however, I don't see much need in you spending the time learning how to pronounce or spell the names of these different classes of medications.

These long, technical, difficult to pronounce names can be intimidating for patients and could use some simplification, making them more user friendly. That is what I would like to do here. It is not necessary to learn everything there is to know about all of these classes of medications and the medications within the classes, just the ones that pertain to you. You do need to know what class of medications the medication you are taking falls into, the name of the medication, what the medication looks like, how much you are supposed to take, when to take the medication and what the side effects are. In fact, you need to know this information for every medication you take whether it is a diabetes medication or not. A really good source for this information is your pharmacist. Not only is a lot of this information given to you in printed form when you pick up your prescriptions, but any questions you have that cannot be answered by reading the enclosed information can usually be answered by the pharmacist. Just be sure to ask!

Too many patients, I have found, take a lot of medicine, however, can not tell me what each medicine is for and what the possible side effects are. And, in fact, if the pill were placed in their hand, they could not tell me its name. That's not good. That is scary. My feeling on this is that if you don't know what you are taking and why you are taking it, you need to find out.

Of the seven classes of oral diabetes medications currently available today, there are three classes that seem to be prescribed most often. I can't say why for sure, but I believe it is probably because doctors have found that when using these classes of medications, either alone or in combination, their patients have had more favorable results than with the other classes of medications. With the continued introduction of newer medications to the market, however, I think this will inevitably change. When I started teaching back in 1993 there were only sulfonylureas and insulin. Now, fifteen years later, six new classes of diabetes medications have been introduced. The availability of these new medications is partly responsible for patients are now living longer and with fewer complications from diabetes.

The three most frequently prescribed classes of oral diabetes medications I am referring to are the sulfonylureas, biguanides and thiozolidinediones. I refer to these as the cheerleaders, security guards and construction crew workers, respectively. In order to understand why I have given each these names, it is necessary to review the three major problems contributing to type 2 diabetes.

Insulin resistance is where it all starts. If you remember from earlier, the inability of the muscle, fat and liver cells to respond to insulin as they should causes the beta cells in the pancreas to produce increasing amounts of insulin over time, eventually leading to the beta cells becoming so overworked and fatigued that they quit working. In my explanation of this I said the hinges on the doors to the muscle, fat and liver cells became rusty, making the doors harder to open. As the rust on the hinges worsened over time, the beta cells were forced to make more and more insulin in order to get the doors open and the glucose in to the cell. To restate, insulin resistance is the first problem. The doors to the muscle, fat and liver cells become too hard to open with normal amounts of insulin, necessitating the need for the beta cells to manufacture increasing quantities of insulin as the insulin resistance continues or worsens over time.

This leads to the second problem, beta cell fatigue and failure, when increasing numbers of beta cells start becoming dysfunctional as a result of having to work so hard to make the necessary insulin. The phase of insulin <u>over production</u> that immediately preceded diabetes is now over, followed by a period now of insulin <u>under production</u>. As beta cell dysfunction continues and less and less insulin is produced and released into the bloodstream, this allows for the manifestation of the third problem, sugar leaking from the liver into the blood. (Remember, one function of the liver is to store excess sugar until a time when it is needed.)

Table 9 - Diabetes Medications

Nickname/How it works	Professional Name	Brand Name	Generic name
Construction Crew Workers	Thiozolidinediones	Avandia	Rosiglitazone

Taking this medication is like sending a crew of construction workers to all of the cells that have rusty hinges, where workers will sand some of the rust off of the hinges and then spray them with WD-40

		Actos	Pioglitazone

Cheerleaders

Taking this medication is like sending a squad of cheerleaders down to the pancreas where they surround the still functioning beta cells and begin to cheer them on, hoping to motivate the beta cells to make more insulin.

Sulfonylureas	Micronase	Glyburide
	Diabeta	
	Glynase	
	Glucotrol	Glipizide
	Glucotrol XL	
	Amaryl	Glimeperide

Cheerleader wannabe's

Not a cheerleader, but does stimulate the production of insulin from beta cells in response to rising glucose levels such as occurs immediately following a meal. Works fast and does not stay in the system as long as a cheerleader.

Meglitinides and	Prandin	Repaglinide
Phenylalinine derivatives	Starlix	Nateglinide

Security Guards

Biguanides	Glucophage	Metformin
	Glucophage XR	

When you take this medicine, it is like sending a detail of security guards to the liver where they will post themselves outside each door to the liver, preventing glucose from leaving the liver and reentering the bloodstream.

Fortamet

Riomet

Multitasking drugs

Incretin mimetics	Byetta Januvia	Exenatide
Gliptins		Sitagliptin

These medications either mimic two naturally occurring hormones that are in short supply in patients with type 2 diabetes (incretin and mimetics), or increase the availability

of these hormones in the blood (gliptins). These medications do several things. They can make you feel full so you won't eat as much, keep your liver from dumping glucose into your blood when you do not need it, and stimulate your beta cells to make insulin when your blood glucose levels are high. Additionally, exenatide slows the rate at which food and glucose leave the stomach.

Carbohydrate blockers

Alpha- Glucosidase	Precose Glyset	Acarbose
Inhibitors		Miglitol

These medications slow the breakdown of carbohydrates in the intestines by competitive inhibition. This results in a reduction in blood glucose levels.

"No seconds, for me"   Amylin Analogs   Symlin   Pramlintide

This medication slows the rate at which food leaves the stomach, prolonging the feeling of fullness. This results in glucose entering the bloodstream more slowly and a lower peak in mealtime blood glucose levels.

Thiozolidinediones - The Construction Crew Workers

Rosiglitazone (Avandia)

Pioglitazone (Actos)

To address the first problem, insulin resistance, we have the construction crew workers, the class of medications typically referred to as thiozolidinediones. These medications improve blood glucose control by traveling to the muscle, fat and liver cells and doing some repair work on the rusty hinges. Every time a construction crew medication is taken it's like sanding some of the rust off of the hinges and spraying them with WD-40, thus making the doors easier to open so the glucose can enter. Construction crew medications target the cells where there is insulin resistance; therefore, they work at the root of the problem, the problem usually leading to type 2 diabetes. Hence, this class of medications improves (or decreases) insulin resistance. (94,95) Repairing rusty hinges is a painstakingly slow process, so it takes at least a couple of weeks to start seeing results after initiating this medication.

Taking one of these medications alone is not likely to cause hypoglycemia because it has no effect on stimulating the manufacture and release of insulin from the beta cells in the pancreas, however, when taken in combination with some of the other classes of diabetes medications may contribute to hypoglycemia. Although medications in this class of drugs have proven very effective for many patients with type 2 diabetes, they are not without risks and are not for everyone. As with all medications patients should read and follow all directions and warnings pertaining to the use of thiozolidinediones before starting to use them. As an example, patients with known kidney and liver problems should not take these medications. Water retention, edema, (the ankles swelling), and increasing body fat mass are all possible side effects. There are additional risks when taking thiozolidinediones that can be found in the literature accompanying the medication.

Sulfonylureas: The Cheerleaders

Chlorpropamide (Diabenese)

Glyburide (Diabeta, Micronase, Glynase)

Glucotrol (Glipizide)

Glimeperide (Amaryl)

One of the problems associated with insulin resistance is that it frequently leads to beta cell failure. The insulin resistance creates a need for the beta cells to step up production of insulin to unusually high levels, eventually causing many of the beta cells to become exhausted and ultimately dysfunctional. The remaining beta cells are still functioning, making insulin, but their production may be falling as they are getting quite tired themselves. This is when doctors frequently prescribe "cheerleader medications" also known as sulfonylureas.

Think of what a cheerleader does. A cheerleader's job is to encourage, motivate, or fire up a crowd. The idea being that if the crowd gets excited and noisy, it will motivate the team to work harder and, as a result, do a little bit better. When taking 5mg. of a cheerleader medication it's like sending 5 cheerleaders down to the pancreas to encourage, motivate and fire up the remaining tired, overworked, beta cells. With encouragement, the expectation is that the beta cells will increase insulin production, resulting in more insulin becoming available to get more cell doors open and more glucose into the cells.

The cheerleader class of medications (sulfonylureas) is relatively inexpensive and usually provides good results, at least for a while. For most patients, the dosage of these medications will usually need to be increased every so often as their effectiveness tends to decline over time. After all, if you saw the same cheerleaders doing the same cheers day after day, month after month, you would eventually tire of them as well. The beta cells work much the same way. Dosages can be increased as necessary until the maximum dose is reached.

Since cheerleader medications stimulate the release of insulin from beta cells, there is always the risk of having a hypoglycemic reaction when taking them, particularly if meals are delayed, skipped, or only a very small amount of carbohydrate is eaten at mealtime. (96) Additionally, if too much exercise is performed without taking the appropriate precautions (checking blood glucose levels before starting to exercise and then eating a small snack if blood glucose levels are not sufficiently high to allow for the normal drop in blood glucose expected to occur with exercise), hypoglycemia can result with this type of medication. It is usually recommended that medications in this class be taken 30 minutes before meals to allow the cheerleaders time to get the beta cells motivated to make more insulin by the time glucose levels start rising after the meal. Weight gain can occur when taking a cheerleader medication because once the insulin delivers the glucose to the various muscle, fat and liver cells throughout the body, if the glucose is not used as a fuel source it will be converted to fat and stored. This is far less likely to happen if the patient is active and exercises regularly.

Biguanides: The Security Guards

Metformin (Glucophage)

As for the third problem, the sugar leaking from the liver into the blood, there is a class of medications for this too. The official name for this class of medications is biguanides; however, I refer to them as the security guards. When there is insufficient insulin circulating in the blood stream, as is usually the case with diabetes, glucose stored in the liver will escape, making its way into the bloodstream and raising blood glucose levels.

Patients frequently ask me why their blood glucose level is higher in the morning than when they went to bed the night before without having had anything to eat. I tell them that in many cases it is because glucose is leaving, or escaping, from their liver and entering their bloodstream while they sleep. In fact, the liver may release the greatest quantity of glucose just before dawn in response to specific hormones released by other parts of the body.

Anytime glucose can escape from the liver and get into the bloodstream that is what it's going to do. Quite frankly, the glucose would much rather be in the bloodstream than in the liver. The problem the glucose has, though, is that when there are normal amounts of insulin in the blood, glucose has a much harder time escaping from the liver. The presence of insulin, particularly normal levels of insulin, has an inhibitory effect on the ability of the glucose to escape from the liver. In the case of most patients with type 2 diabetes, there is frequently too little insulin circulating in the blood, which allows the glucose to successfully escape from the liver and enter the bloodstream, thereby raising the blood glucose level.

Metformin, a security guard medication, works by reducing the amount of glucose that escapes from the liver. As an example, if 500mg. of metformin are taken before bed, it's like sending 500 security guards to the liver to stand guard outside each door to the liver. Then when glucose tries to open a door and sneak out, headed for the blood, the security guard can foil the escape by quickly closing the door, keeping the sugar safely contained inside the liver.

It is important to understand that it is completely normal for glucose to be inside the liver as it is one of the liver's many functions to store glucose. It is not an abnormality caused by having type 2 diabetes. During times of physical or mental stress the liver is supposed to release some of the stored sugar back into the bloodstream. The problem with this for patients with type 2 diabetes is that when some of the glucose is released back into the blood stream there is an insufficient amount of insulin available in the blood to pick up the glucose and carry it where it needs to go. In the person without diabetes, anytime the level of glucose in the blood starts dropping, before it can get uncomfortably low, the liver releases some of its stored glucose back into the bloodstream, maintaining normal blood glucose levels. This particular function of the liver that actually serves as a safety net for the person without diabetes can, unfortunately, be quite a problem for the person with type 2 diabetes.

Besides metformin's primary role as a security guard, this medication plays a lesser secondary role as a construction crew worker, doing repair work on the rusty hinges, helping the doors to the cells open easier. Unlike the construction crew and cheerleader medications, metformin, does not cause weight gain; in fact, a small weight loss of 2-5kgs may actually occur once treatment with metformin is initiated. (96)

In addition to metformin's ability to reduce the flow of glucose from the liver into the bloodstream, it can have a very favorable effect on the lipid or fat content circulating in the blood. Triglycerides, LDL's and total cholesterol levels in the blood have been shown to drop when using metformin, while simultaneously raising the good HDL cholesterol. (97, 98) This is a real plus, considering that elevated or abnormal blood lipid levels are so common in patients with diabetes. Since metformin does not stimulate the release of insulin from the beta cells, when used alone it is not likely to produce hypoglycemia. Metformin needs to be taken with food to minimize the likelihood of stomach distress, nausea, diarrhea, etc., and should not be used in patients with kidney or liver disease.

Combination Medications

Glucovance

Metaglip

Avandamet

Actoplusmet

Avandaryl

Duetact

Janumet

It is becoming more and more common for physicians to prescribe more than one class of medications early in the course of a patient's diabetes, maybe not with the onset of diabetes, but within several months. With this in mind, several years ago, pharmaceutical companies thought there might be benefit in combining certain classes of medications. A major benefit would be improved compliance, that is, by combining two different diabetes medications into one pill there would be fewer pills to take, or fewer pills to forget to take.

Initially the cheerleader medications were combined with security guard medications, glyburide with metformin (Glucovance), and glipizide with metformin (Metaglip). Then construction crew medications were combined with a security guard medication, rosiglitazone with metformin (Avandamet) and pioglitozone with metformin (Actoplusmet). More recently a cheerleader medication was combined with construction crew medications, glimiperide with rosiglitazone (Avandaryl) and glimiperide with pioglitozone

(Duetact). The newest of the combination medications is called Janumet, a combination of the incretin mimetic sitagliptin with metformin.

It is important for patients to remember that not only will they derive the benefits of each of the contributing medications that make up the combination drug, but they will also need to pay attention to the precautions, side effects and contraindications of each contributing medication as if they were taking it separately.

If we look into the future, I wouldn't be surprised to see more combination medications on the way and, eventually, all three classes of medications, the cheerleaders, security guards and construction crew workers, being combined.

Meglitinides and Phenylalanine Derivatives

Repaglinide (Prandin)

Nateglinide (Starlix)

I didn't nickname this class of medications but can tell you they behave similarly to the cheerleader medications in that they stimulate the release of insulin. Both medications, repaglinide (Prandin) and nateglinide (Starlix), do basically the same thing, the only difference between the two being their derivation. Repaglinide is derived from benzoic acid, which makes it a meglitinide, while nateglinide is derived from D-phenylalanine, making it a phenylalanine derivative. These medications work very quickly, enhancing the release of insulin from the beta cells of the pancreas but only when glucose levels are high, such as after eating, similar to the way beta cells release insulin after eating in a person without diabetes. (99) Since these medications only exert their influence when blood glucose levels are high, and because they are only active for approximately three hours, the possibility of hypoglycemic reactions is reduced, making them safer than the cheerleader medications. (100,101)

With cheerleader medications, the ability to stimulate insulin production is dependent on the amount of the medication taken, that is to say the greater the dose taken the more insulin likely to be produced. With repaglinide and nateglinide it is the level of sugar (glucose) in the blood that determines how much insulin the beta cells produce and release.

There is risk of hypoglycemia with these two medications, however, to a much lesser degree than with cheerleader medications.

Alpha-Glucosidase Inhibitors

Acarbose (Precose)

Miglitol (Glycet)

The idea behind this class of medications sounds good and the two medications in this class, Acarbose and Miglitol, would probably be prescribed more often if it weren't for the troubling side effects many patients experience when taking either of these medications. This class of medications works by inhibiting certain enzymes that are involved in carbohydrate digestion. This results in a reduction in the amount of carbohydrate absorbed and prevents the blood sugar from climbing as high after meals. (96)

The downside of this are the gastrointestinal side effects frequently encountered, including diarrhea and flatulence. Regardless of how well the medication is working, I have noticed that many patients often do not continue with the treatment as they feel the side effects outweigh the benefits.

Until the gastrointestinal disturbances can be minimized, I believe it is doubtful this medication will be widely used.

Amylin Analogs

Pramlintide (Symlin)

To keep things as simple as possible and to help patients better understand their diabetes, I tell them in class that insulin is made in the beta cells and that making insulin is the only thing the beta cells do. I have recently started modifying my comments to say that insulin is one of two hormones the beta cells produce. Beta cells also produce another hormone known as amylin, a naturally occurring hormone that is co-secreted with insulin. (102) Amylin also plays a role in blood sugar control and is lacking in type 1 and type 2 diabetes. (103) Pramlintide is a synthetic analogue of human amylin that was produced to have the same action as amylin. Pramlintide, the generic form of the medication designed to replace amylin in amylin deficient patients, helps control blood sugar levels differently than medications discussed so far. Pramlintide slows the rate of gastric emptying and increases feelings of satiety. (104) In other words, it slows down the rate at which food leaves your stomach and makes you feel satisfied or less hungry. As a result, there is a reduced peak in post meal blood sugar levels, and you end up eating less, which promotes weight loss.

By inhibiting another hormone known as glucagon, Pramlintide also reduces the amount of sugar that is released from the liver and enters the blood. This also contributes to overall Improvement in blood sugar control. With the exception of causing the liver to release less sugar into the blood, this medication does indeed control blood sugar levels by actions not discussed previously. Several precautions need to be taken when taking this medication to avoid the potentially serious side effect of having a severe low blood glucose reaction. Pramlinitide cannot be mixed with insulin and should not be taken if skipping a meal or eating fewer than 250 calories. Also, mealtime insulin dosages need to be reduced typically 30-50 percent when the medication is first started. (105) As always, patients should read the medication literature that accompanies the medication and follow all precautionary measures.

Incretin Mimetics

Exenatide (Byetta)

Research has shown that more insulin is produced when glucose or sugar enters the body through oral ingestion versus when similar amounts of glucose are infused intravenously.

This phenomenon has been called the "incretin-effect" which has led researchers to believe that there is something going on in the gastrointestinal tract that influences insulin production. (106,107,108) GLP-1 and GIP are two incretin hormones that have been found to stimulate insulin production and contribute to the achievement of normal blood sugar levels after meals. (109) Both hormones, GLP-1 and GIP, stimulate glucose dependent increased insulin production and slow the emptying of food from the stomach. (110,111, 112) GLP-1 also suppresses glucagon production, a hormone that acts in opposition to insulin and increases the amount of sugar in the blood via the liver, promotes a feeling of satiety, leads to eating less food and, therefore, weight loss. (111,112,113)

Based on this information, a new class of medications has emerged known as incretin-mimetics. The first medication in this class to be approved by the Food and Drug Administration is Exenatide. This medication acts much the same as the naturally produced GLP-1, in that it stimulates glucose-dependent insulin release, restricts the flow of sugar from the liver by inhibiting the action of glucagon, slows the rate at which food leaves the stomach therefore slowing the rate at which sugar enters the blood thus avoiding high peaks in blood sugar after meals, and decreases appetite leading to weight loss.

Exenatide has to be injected just like insulin; however, it is presently only available in a pen. It is not available in a vial to be drawn up in a syringe and injected.

As for possible side effects, hypoglycemia has been reported when exenatide is combined with a cheerleader medication, (sulfonylurea) or a cheerleader medicine plus a security guard medication (metformin). Aside from hypoglycemia, gastrointestinal disorders such as nausea, vomiting and diarrhea are the most common side effects that likely will diminish over time.

Gliptins (DPP-4 inhibitors)

Sitigliptin (Januvia)

Vildagliptin (Galvus)

The gliptins, commonly referred to as DPP-4 inhibitors, are the newest class of medications being used to treat type 2 diabetes. Sitigliptin (Januvia) improves blood glucose control in two ways: it increases insulin production by the beta cells when needed and decreases the amount of glucose dumped into the blood by the liver. (114) It accomplishes this by blocking the action of DPP-4, an enzyme responsible for limiting GLP-1 and GIP in circulation. When GLP-1 and GIP are limited, less insulin is produced by the beta cells and more glucose is released from the liver to enter the blood. This medication works in an insulin dependent manner; that is, it only causes an increase in insulin production by the beta cells if the blood glucose level is elevated. Additionally, there does not appear to be the associated weight gain with sitigliptin that is so commonly found with the cheerleader medications (sulfonylureas) and construction crew workers (thiozolidinediones), nor the increased risk of hypoglycemia, low blood glucose, associated with the cheerleader medications (sulfonylureas). I like to think of sitagliptin and the rest of the gliptin family as the result of a marriage between a cheerleader medication and a security guard drug.

To Clarify . . . Sometimes people get the Incretin mimetics and Gliptins (DPP4 inhibitors) confused. Just remember that incretin mimetics mimic, or do nearly the same thing as naturally produced incretins and that there is a reduction in incretin production with type 2 diabetes. By injecting an incretin mimetic you help restore the desired incretin effect. Gliptins will increase the level of naturally produced incretins by blocking the action of DPP-4, a substance known to limit the amount of incretins circulating in the blood.

Adjusting Medication on Your Own

To put it very simply, don't do it. Don't make any adjustments to your diabetes medication regimen without first discussing it with your doctor.

There have been far too many instances when, after checking a patient's blood sugar and finding it to be a bit high, the patient has responded with, "I quit taking one of my diabetes medications a couple of days ago, and I wondered how that was going to affect my blood sugar. Do you think I should start taking it again? Or, "I'm doing an experiment this week and not taking any of my diabetes medications to see what it will do to my blood glucose levels. I know it's a little high now, but it was only 118mg/dl. this morning. I guess that means I may not need the evening pill. What do you think?"

I think that it is a big mistake to make adjustments to your diabetes medication regimen or any medication. It's dangerous and therefore should not be done. If patients have questions regarding their medications, they should bring these questions to their doctor.

If a medication change is necessary, for whatever reason, the doctor, PA, or ARNP should be the one to make the change. If the change is desired because the patient feels the current medication regimen is not adequate, the doctor will usually want the patient to check their blood glucose levels four to six times a day for several days prior to the appointment so the doctor can review the numbers to see what has been going on.

When a patient is on insulin therapy, it is common for a doctor to put the patient on what is called a "sliding scale." This means a patient will follow a predetermined scale established by the doctor that describes how much insulin should be taken depending on the patient's blood glucose level. Sliding scales may be quite appropriate for some patients requiring insulin and not at all appropriate for others. Only when a patient's doctor has given the patient instructions as to how to adjust their insulin themselves, or has given them a sliding scale, should the patient do so. Insulin is very potent and taking more than needed is likely to result in low blood sugar levels or hypoglycemia. When blood glucose levels go low, it is unpleasant to say the least, but when they go really low, it can be dangerous and even fatal.

Chapter 8
Insulin

As mentioned previously, it is generally thought that everyone with type 2 diabetes will eventually end up taking insulin if they have the disease for a long enough period of time, due to the progressive nature of the illness. The gradual decline in insulin production resulting from steadily increasing beta cell dysfunction is thought to continue indefinitely, and with present knowledge, the best a patient can hope for is to slow the process. Although currently there are no studies that indicate exercise will slow the process, or better yet, stop the process, it is promising that the initiation of exercise in a previously sedentary patient can lead to, and has many times lead to a reduction in the amount of medication required, sometimes to the point of eliminating the medication altogether.

Perhaps exercise is helping to preserve the remaining beta cells, or maybe with exercise the patient simply needs a lot less insulin, an amount the patient may still be able to make. Regardless of the reason, a reduction in the need for medication with exercise is a promising approach. Research designed specifically to look at whether exercise can postpone or eliminate the need for ultimately ever having to take insulin injections is lacking and needs to be done. If future research proves what I think it will, that the performance of regular exercise can delay or permanently postpone the need for a patient to start on insulin injections, then the argument for exercise becomes even stronger than it already is and, hopefully, will encourage more physicians to promote exercise with greater enthusiasm.

Insulin therapy is usually recommended to patients when the maximal dose of oral medications is not effective at controlling blood glucose levels. Once a doctor says it's time to initiate insulin, I suggest you don't resist. Doctor avoidance, that is, canceling or missing doctor appointments because you are afraid the doctor is going to recommend you start insulin therapy, could be a very, very costly mistake. Many patients try to bargain or plead with the doctor to avoid or postpone initiating insulin therapy. That's something you probably don't want to do. Not taking insulin when the time comes when you need it, probably because oral medications are no longer controlling blood glucose levels, will likely result in higher blood glucose levels and higher HbA1C, thus leading to microvascular complications, or a worsening of them if they are already present. This could be very dangerous.

It is very helpful and important to have the right attitude when beginning insulin therapy.

Patients could look at starting insulin therapy as a new beginning, a new option that may help them control their diabetes more effectively and more easily than with oral medications. I have known patients who found it a relief to start using insulin because they were finally able to achieve better blood sugar control, particularly if they had been struggling with oral medications over a long period of time. Sometimes the physician will simply say it's time to start insulin because the oral medications are no longer effective, enroll the patient in an insulin initiation class and three days later the patient is using insulin.

There are other times, and I have heard this frequently, when the physician tells the patient that they have three months to get their blood glucose levels under better control or they will be started on insulin. This doesn't always sit well with the patient as many times the patient feels they are being threatened or punished for not taking better care of their diabetes.

I cannot begin to know what a physician's motives are for making this threatening statement; however, I do have some ideas. In some cases it seems to have served as a wake up call. I have seen patients finally enroll and participate in a comprehensive diabetes management class; something the doctor may have been encouraging for a long time. Patients have become motivated to improve their eating habits and even start an exercise program. I have had many patients enroll in my exercise program as a last resort, hoping to avoid taking insulin. Could this be the reason the physician said what he did? Was it meant by the physician to be a wake up call, an attempt by the physician to get the patient to take a more active roll in their diabetes care?

Often times after talking with a patient and perhaps looking over their logbooks the physician can get a pretty good idea of how hard patients are working to control their diabetes. If the patient's blood sugars are out of control, and the physician believes the patient can do a lot better, the physician may give the patient three months to improve before initiating insulin and try to motivate the patient that way. This may prove very effective, particularly if the physician knows the patient is opposed to taking insulin. The physician may feel that with improved effort by the patient, the blood sugars may improve enough that insulin may not be necessary after the three months.

Patients need to hear from the doctor that allowing them to remain on oral medications when they are no longer controlling the blood sugar levels would lead to the onset of diabetic complications. Even when this is explained, the patient doesn't always "hear" or get the meaning of what the doctor is saying.

Every effort should always be made to control a patient's diabetes with as little medication as possible. Ideally, only when improved eating habits and exercise alone fail to adequately control blood glucose levels, should medications of any sort be initiated. Patients should never rely exclusively on medications to keep their blood glucose levels under good control with little regard to what they are eating and how much they are exercising.

When It's Time to Start Insulin

When the time comes to start taking insulin, if it does come, and for many it will, it would be wise to get some formal instruction on how to best get started. Now don't get the wrong idea, it is not difficult, in fact there is not much to it, once you know how to do it. Giving the injection incorrectly, or knowing little or nothing about the type of insulin you take, its precautions and how it works, can be very dangerous. Undoubtedly, there will be many questions before giving the first injection, all of which should be answered by a certified diabetes educator, if possible. I suggest a certified diabetes educator because they are the best qualified to provide instruction on everything you need to know when initiating insulin therapy.

Apprehension before the injection: The fear of injecting themselves with a syringe sometimes two to three times a day is the cause of great apprehension in many patients faced with starting insulin therapy. Although I am not in a position to experience everything someone with diabetes must go through, I can sympathize to some degree, at least when it comes to injections.

When I was about twelve years old, I was told I would have to start taking allergy shots three days a week. Well, for me, at that age, I thought it was about the worst thing that could happen. How could I ever enjoy anything again knowing that I was going to get a shot at what basically amounted to every other day! Granted, when we're twelve most of us are pretty naïve of really serious hardships, at least I was. Back then I got sick with bronchitis at least several times each winter and hated going to the doctor because he always gave me a shot in the upper arm, and that hurt a lot. I thought if I tightened the muscle in my arm it wouldn't hurt as much. Boy was I wrong! In fact, I was wrong about the whole idea of getting allergy shots.

First of all, my doctor always gave me my antibiotics in my shoulder muscle, also known as the deltoid. It was an intramuscular injection, meaning the needle was injected directly into the muscle, and the needle was at least twice as long as the one they would use on me at the allergy doctor. The allergist would be giving me my injections subcutaneously, which means just below the skin where there is a little bit of fat. Shorter needle length translated to much less pain. The allergist also told me to stop flexing the muscles in my arm and the shot would hurt less. Why didn't my pediatrician tell me this? Well, as it turned out, having to get allergy shots for several years was no big deal at all. It didn't hurt. I was so relieved after getting my first injection. The anxiety I had experienced leading up to that first injection was totally unnecessary. Over the years I have taught many patients about insulin and how to inject it. Some of the comments I have heard immediately following a patient's first injection follow.

"Is that it, I didn't hardly feel it?"

"Is that all there is to it; that's not bad at all. That didn't even hurt?"

"Oh, I can do this, there is nothing to it; heck, pricking my finger to test my blood sugar is worse than this."

I have heard that comment many, many times. I can honestly say that of those patients I have taught who were apprehensive about giving themselves injections, they were all very relieved and confident in their ability to give future injections.

When the apprehension of giving the injection is gone, patients are ready to learn about the kind of insulin they will be taking and the source from which it came. There are many kinds of insulin and the time frame in which they start to work, the time they work at peak effectiveness, and the period of time that they exert their blood glucose lowering effect differ dramatically. This will all be discussed in the next several sections.

The Need for Insulin

In the early 1920's, when insulin was first administered to type 1 patients, it saved lives. Prior to this, when exogenous insulin was not available, patients diagnosed with type 1 could not survive more than several months. It's now typical for a patient with type 1 diabetes, to inject usually two to four times per day. Without daily injections of insulin, it would be impossible to control blood glucose levels regardless of what was eaten and how much exercise was performed. In addition, muscle, fat and liver cells would starve as other nutrients and energy sources in the blood, such as protein and fat, could not get into the cells to nourish them either. The patient would become malnourished even though he or she may have been eating everything in sight. Eventually this would lead to the malnourished cells trying to derive energy by breaking down (metabolizing) stored fat. This may not seem like a bad thing, but I assure you that it can be very dangerous, particularly for someone with diabetes. It all comes down to this: When processes in the body metabolize fat for the purposes of making energy, glucose must be broken down at the same time. In other words, glucose is necessary for the proper metabolism of fat.

If no glucose can leave the blood and enter the cells as a result of having no insulin, as is the case with a patient with untreated type1, the cells have no energy source and in desperation will begin to metabolize fat as a potential fuel source. In the process, however, an undesirable byproduct of incomplete fat metabolism is generated that is referred to as a ketone body. If ketones are allowed to accumulate in the blood due to prolonged periods of incomplete fat metabolism, a patient with type 1 diabetes could develop a condition known as diabetic ketoacidosis or DKA, a very serious and potentially life threatening condition.

When in class, I sometimes ask patients if any of them have ever made cookies or cakes before. Of those that say they have, I ask them what ingredient is needed, but in very small quantities, to make the recipe turn out the way it is supposed to? Vanilla extract!

When younger, I was always mystified by the way my mom could take a small taste of cookie dough, move it around in her mouth for a few seconds and then tell me it was missing something. "It needs just a little more vanilla," or "I know what I did, I forgot to add the vanilla," she would tell me. Although the recipe only called for a very small amount of vanilla, the finished product would not taste, as it should if the vanilla were left out. The same can be said for glucose. Although not much glucose is required, proper fat metabolism cannot proceed, as it should without glucose being present.

This is why type 1 patients must always take their prescribed dose of insulin without interruption. The longer a type 1 patient goes between prescribed insulin injections the greater the likelihood of elevated blood glucose readings and, eventually, diabetic ketoacidosis.

Note: In type 1 patients, performing regular exercise usually reduces the need for as much insulin, however, it never does eliminate the need for it altogether.

The History of Insulin

Insulin was discovered in 1921 by Banting and Best. (115,116) This doctor and medical student were able to successfully isolate and extract insulin from the pancreas of a dog.

The following year, in 1922, insulin was first used to treat a patient with type 1 diabetes. (115)

Over the next sixty years or so insulin was acquired from porcine or bovine sources and was frequently referred to as beef or pork insulin. It was also referred to as "regular insulin." During this time modifications were continually made to regular insulin that would change its performance characteristics, making it more applicable for human use. In 1936, Protamine, a protein obtained from the sperm of fish, and zinc were added to regular insulin. These additions slowed the action of the insulin and delayed its blood glucose lowering effect. (116) Continued experimentation with different formulations of insulin resulted in the development of NPH in 1938 and Lente in 1952, both considered intermediate acting insulin. Both of these insulin were slower to start working than regular insulin, peaked much later than regular insulin, and stayed in the blood stream longer.

Although beef and pork insulin were successfully used for years, many people unfortunately suffered from the unpleasant side effect of allergic reactions. These reactions usually manifested themselves as irritations to the skin at the injection site. (96) Since these were the only kinds of insulin available back then, patients had to either stop taking the insulin, which was obviously not an option, or tolerate the allergic reactions.

Fortunately, particularly for those patients having allergic reactions to insulin obtained from animals, a researcher by the name of Sanger was able to determine the amino acid sequence of human insulin in 1955. This led to the genetic engineering of the first synthetic "human insulin" in 1983, insulin that for the vast majority of patients did not produce allergic reactions. (115) At first glance you might think human insulin comes from, well, humans. But despite its name, this insulin does not come from a human pancreas. Human insulin is a biosynthetic insulin that comes from the bacteria, E.Coli, or from fungal cells known as Saccharomyces cerevisiae. (96)

Almost ten years later, in 1992, genetic engineering gave rise to the first insulin analog known as lispro. (116) An insulin analog is insulin where the amino acid sequence has been altered in some way to change the performance characteristics of the insulin. In the case of insulin lispro the manipulation of the amino acid sequence resulted in a much faster acting insulin than had been available previously.

In the case of glargine, an insulin analog introduced shortly after insulin lispro, it was the first insulin analog that closely mimicked the basal secretions of normal beta cells. (117) In a person without diabetes, the beta cells are never totally resting; they are always producing a small amount of insulin. In a sense it's as if all the beta cells have leaky faucets, in that even when turned off there are always drops of insulin entering the bloodstream. "Basal insulins" as these long acting "peakless" insulin analogs are referred to, ensure there is a low level of insulin circulating in the blood stream 24 hours a day.

Types of Insulin

Patients requiring insulin today have a wide variety of insulin to choose from. These insulins range from those that exert their blood glucose lowering influence very quickly and then are finished working, to those that exert their blood glucose lowering effect to a much lesser degree but over a much longer period of time. In order to develop insulin with such varying characteristics it was necessary to physically manipulate the molecular structure of the insulin by rearranging or replacing gene sequences or by adding agents (buffers) to the insulin to slow down its blood glucose lowering effect.

People with diabetes now have the capability to control their diabetes better than ever before due in large part to advances in medication including insulin. With careful strategic planning, usually worked out by the doctor, or the diabetes care team, made up of the doctor, CDE nurse educator, CDE dietician and patient, the right amount, of the right type, or types of insulin, taken at the right time, should keep the blood sugar levels pretty well controlled. This is assuming that the patient is eating reasonably well and getting plenty of physical activity.

Regular Insulin

The insulin obtained from the pancreas of animals had to be purified before it was ready for injection into humans. The finished, purified product was clear and colorless. When it was injected, assuming it was pure, the time it took to start working after injection could be estimated. The period of time when it exerted its greatest effect on blood glucose levels could be estimated. Even the total length of time it was effective in lowering blood glucose levels could be estimated.

I use the word, "estimated" because there are various circumstances that that either speed up or slow down the action of the insulin after its injection. This can be problematic if the insulin peaks sooner or later than it is predicted to, or if it remains in the bloodstream longer than is expected. This could result in blood glucose levels that are either too high or too low. Regular insulin, as it was called, was the fastest working insulin available. It was "estimated" to start exerting its blood glucose lowering effect as soon as 30-60 minutes after injection; however, regular insulin peaked, or was most effective, two to three hours after injection and had a total duration of action of four to six hours. (118) For this insulin to be most effective, it is recommended it be taken about 30-45 minutes before each meal.

Buffered Insulin

As already mentioned in the history of insulin, in the 1930's buffers were added to regular insulin to change its behavior characteristics. Intermediate acting insulins such as PZI, an abbreviation for Protamine zinc insulin, NPH insulin, an abbreviation for Neutral Protamine Hagedorn, and Lente were created. They are referred to as intermediate acting insulins. Lente insulin, however, tends to work a little longer than the NPH. (118) Buffers are responsible for slowing the insulin's start time, delaying the time period when the insulin peaks and lengthening its duration of action.

Ultralente is considered a long acting insulin containing still more buffer. To give an idea of the effect manipulating the amount of buffer has on the insulin, NPH and Lente, intermediate acting insulins, start working 2-4 hours after injection, peak 4-8 hours after injection, and have a duration of action that lasts for 10-20 hours. (118)

Ultralente starts to work 6-10 hours after injection, doesn't really have a peak and has a duration of action that lasts 20-30 hours. (118)

Doctors often take advantage of the various peak times of the different insulins and sometimes prescribe two different insulins with different peak times be mixed in the same syringe and be taken in the morning before breakfast and just before dinner. As an example, if regular insulin that peaks 2-3 hours after being injected were taken in the morning, 30 minutes before breakfast, along with an intermediate acting insulin that peaks 4-8 hours after injection, it is conceivable that no other insulin would need to be taken until mid to late afternoon when both insulins have finished peaking and their effect on blood glucose levels is starting to wane. In summary, the addition of buffered insulins has enabled many patients to successfully control their diabetes with fewer injections.

Insulin Analogs

Quick Acting

Lispro (Humalog)

Aspart (Novolog)

Glulisine (Apidra)

Another way to alter insulin's behavior characteristics is to change its physical structure. By slightly rearranging the amino acid sequence of the insulin, or substituting one amino acid for another, manufacturers found they could create insulin that begins to work much faster than regular insulin and also an insulin that works for a very long period of time and has no peak to its action. Insulins created by manipulating the amino acids in some way are called insulin analogs.

There are now three insulin analogs that go to work very quickly after injection and are all basically the same. They are known as insulin lispro, insulin aspart (118) the newest of the three, and insulin glulisine. These insulins can be injected just minutes before a meal and seem to keep postprandial blood glucose levels under better control than when injecting regular insulin 30 minutes before meals. Once injected, these insulins can start working within 15-30 minutes and peak in about 1-2 hours after injection. Approximately

3-5 hours after injection these quick acting insulins have run their course and have little to no effect on future blood glucose levels.

Long Acting

Glargine (Lantus)

Detemir (Levemir)

The first of the long acting insulin analogs to be developed is glargine. It starts working 1-2 hours after injection and has no peak to its action. That is, the effect the insulin has on lowering blood glucose levels 2 or 3 hours after injection is the same as 8-10 hours after injection. It is designed to be a 24 hour insulin, having a blood glucose lowering effect for a full 24 hours. Glargine has been shown to control blood glucose levels with similar effectiveness as NPH when the NPH is injected 1-2 times a day. (117)

Two of the advantages glargine has over NPH insulin, are its ability to control blood glucose levels with less weight gain and a reduced risk of nocturnal hypoglycemia. (119) This is in addition to the fact that it only has to be injected once a day.

The most recent long acting insulin analog introduced to the market is insulin detemir, an analog with a very similar pattern of action as insulin glargine. It has a relatively flat peak and also provides blood glucose control for approximately 24 hours.

Premixed Combination Insulins

Prior to the release of insulin analogs, premixed insulins were often used with patients who wanted the benefits of a fast acting insulin, such as regular, and an intermediate acting insulin, such as NPH, but did not want to take two separate injections.

The first of the premixed insulins was a combination of fast acting regular insulin and intermediate acting NPH insulin. It was known as 70/30. A bottle of 70/30 was made up of 70 percent NPH and 30 percent regular insulin. Although this ratio of insulin would not work for all patients needing mixed insulin, patients already mixing their insulin in similar proportions to what came pre-mixed, sometimes are able to switch to the pre-mixed version. This may not seem to be a big advantage to patients who have no problem giving themselves injections, but for patients who have a hard time seeing the lines and numbers on the syringe and accurately measuring and drawing up their insulin, this is a big deal. Anytime a patient with these problems can reduce the number of times he or she has to draw up and inject themselves, the better.

There are several mixtures of human insulin presently available including the 70/30 insulin, just mentioned, and the 50/50, which is 50 percent NPH and 50 percent regular insulin. More recently, newer fixed combination human insulin analogs have become available. Human insulin analog mix, 75/25, which is 75 percent neutral protamine lispro, NPL, an intermediate acting insulin very similar to NPH, and 25 percent lispro, the insulin that starts to work almost immediately after injection and the other is insulin analog mix 70/30, which is 70 percent neutral protamine aspart, again, with characteristics similar to the NPH, and 30 percent aspart.

As you can well imagine, there is no best insulin or insulin regimen that is most appropriate for all patients. An insulin regimen a patient may have started with, that worked very well for a couple of years, may over the course of the next year or so need to be changed as the patient changes. As an example, let's say the patient gains 20 pounds, or better still, let's say the patient loses 20 pounds! The dose of insulin or type of insulin is likely to change.

Fortunately for physicians and patients alike there are many different kinds of insulin, each with its own characteristics that can be tried until treatment goals are reached.

The determination of which insulin or insulin therapy the physician recommends is based on a number of factors. One very significant factor is how willing the patient is to give more than one injection a day. When the doctor has a highly motivated patient with little anxiety regarding giving injections, that is willing to test blood glucose levels 3-4 or more times per day, the doctor is more likely to prescribe intensive insulin therapy. Patients on intensive insulin therapy will usually take one of the long acting insulins such as glargine or detemir, once a day, usually at night, and a rapid acting insulin analog such as lispro, aspart or glulisine just before meals.

Intensive insulin therapy has been shown to be very effective at maintaining optimal blood glucose levels, thereby reducing the risk of the microvascular complications, neuropathy, retinopathy and nephropathy.

For patients with greater degrees of anxiety, who are injecting themselves, an intensive insulin regimen is usually not appropriate and other insulin therapy regimens are necessary. I have found there are other reasons patients may be unwilling to give multiple daily injections besides the fact that they are fearful of needles. Convenience may be an issue.

As an educator it is important to remember that a patient's unwillingness to give multiple daily injections does not necessarily reflect on the patient's motivation to care for their diabetes.

There are alternative options requiring patients to inject only once or twice per day. In the twice a day scenario the patient may be advised to mix an intermediate acting insulin like NPH with a short acting insulin such as regular and inject that in the morning before breakfast and in the evening before dinner. If the patient's insulin requirements are very similar to one of the premixed insulins, the patient may elect to use one of them, either 70/30 or 50/50, or one of the premixed analogs 75/25 or 70/30. If the patient will only be injecting once per day, then more than likely it will be a long acting, non-peaking insulin analog such as glargine or detemir.

These are examples of what the doctor might recommend, but they are not exhaustive and there are other possible insulin regimens and recommendations regarding insulin use the doctor might make. The examples I have presented are not recommendations as to what a patient should do, but simply examples of what a doctor might recommend to a patient starting on insulin therapy. My examples should not take the place of seeing your doctor for medical care.

Pens vs Syringes

When administering insulin today patients have the option of using either a traditional insulin syringe or an insulin pen. An insulin pen looks like a fatter, longer writing pen complete with a clip so you can attach it to your shirt pocket. When pens were first introduced they came with replaceable 300 unit cartridges that you loaded into the pen and then disposed of when empty. Newer pens are disposable meaning that when the insulin that is preloaded into the pen is used up, the entire pen is discarded. When pen users are ready to give an injection of insulin, they simply take the cap off the pen, screw a needle onto the end of the pen, dial up the prescribed dose, give the injection, unscrew the needle, and put the cap back on the pen.

That's basically it. As with any new device, insulin pen users should read all of the instructions provided with the pen and make sure they understand how to use the pen correctly. My summary here is not intended to teach a patient how to use an insulin pen nor should it take the place of formal instruction regarding insulin pen use.

I will not attempt to instruct in the proper use of either the insulin syringe or the insulin pen as this should be done with the assistance and in the presence of a medical professional such as a nurse, physician or diabetes educator. I would not want anyone to try administering insulin based solely on the information provided in this book.

Chapter 9
Acute Complications and Foot Care

Hypoglycemia

Hypoglycemia (low blood sugar) results when blood glucose levels drop too low and signs and symptoms of low blood glucose are present. A more official definition is a blood glucose level below 100mg/dl. with symptoms. Hypoglycemia is potentially a very dangerous and serious situation that requires immediate attention. Failure to adequately treat severe hypoglycemia could result in death. Failure to treat even moderately low blood glucose levels could have serious consequences if the person tries to drive or perform any task requiring normal levels of concentration or thinking.

One big concern about hypoglycemia is that someone could become hypoglycemic, not recognize the symptoms or know how to properly treat it, and continue about their business. Others nearby may notice the hypoglycemic individual acting somewhat peculiar or inappropriate. They may notice decreased work production, slurring of speech, rude or silly behavior, reckless or careless driving, or the person appearing as if they had too much to drink. Some of this behavior could lead to an accident or injury.

There have been reports on the news and in the papers of someone driving off the road and into a house because of hypoglycemia. One of my patients came to class because he had recently had a car accident; he passed out and ran off the road. He didn't remember this or exactly what happened. He only knew this because sometime later, probably several hours later, when in the emergency room, once his blood glucose level came back up and he was coherent again, someone told him what had happened.

I believe he was ticketed and I do know that his license was taken away. He was a professor at a nearby college. I remember him telling me what an inconvenience it had been not being able to drive. I also recall him telling me all the things he had to go through to get his license reinstated. Apparently, if your license is taken away or suspended for this sort of thing, it is not easy to get it reinstated any time soon. At least it wasn't in this gentleman's case.

There have been cases when people who became severely hypoglycemic have become combative when people have tried to help them such as in the emergency room. I have heard stories of people "waking up" on the floor, and they have no idea how they got there. Sometimes they remember they were trying to get to the kitchen to get something to eat because they could feel their blood sugar going too low. Others believe they must have passed out because their blood sugar was too low, but they don't remember it being low prior to losing consciousness.

I know of one patient who has had numerous car accidents as a result of his blood sugar going too low. This particular person seems to have what has been termed "hypoglycemic unawareness." If someone is to develop hypoglycemic unawareness, it is usually going to be someone who has had diabetes for a long period of time and is no longer aware when the usual hypoglycemic symptoms appear. The early warning system that is built into all of us that tells us when the blood glucose levels are dropping too low is not working as well as it should anymore.

It is also common for these people to have frequent hypoglycemic episodes that seem to worsen the condition. It is not uncommon for someone with hypoglycemic unawareness to be walking around with blood sugars down in the 40mg/dl. range or even lower and not even know it. What makes this so dangerous is that this person, although walking around and seeming to be all right, is really far from it. This person is not likely to be "with it" and is actually probably "out of it." It would be extremely dangerous for this person to attempt driving or to do anything that requires any concentration or thinking. Utilizing power tools, operating equipment or trying to drive anything could be disastrous. Once down this low this person could be just a few points away from losing consciousness.

When a person does lose consciousness due to a severe hypoglycemic episode, this is the result of the brain not getting enough glucose. It is about the same thing as when your car runs out of gas and stops. It can't run without gas. Your brain cannot operate without glucose. Put another way, the only fuel your brain can use is glucose. When the symptoms of low blood glucose first start to appear, that is the same thing as when the yellow warning light comes on in your car in the little gas gauge window. Anytime someone loses consciousness due to hypoglycemia, it is dangerous; after all, it means the brain is severely short on fuel. If treated immediately and properly, the patient should recover without any permanent damage. It has been discussed, however, that a person with frequent hypoglycemic episodes that result in a loss of consciousness may actually be left with some residual damage to brain cells as a result of the chronic deprivation of glucose.

For most people with type 2 diabetes, particularly if they are newly diagnosed or have not had diabetes for a long time, the onset of hypoglycemic symptoms will occur when blood sugar levels drop down to approximately 80mg/dl. Please note that I used the word approximately here because not everyone will feel the symptoms for hypoglycemia at the same blood glucose reading. 80mg/dl. is an approximation only. You may know someone who feels symptoms at 85 or 90mg/dl. or 70-75mg/dl. You may feel symptoms one day at

83mg/dl. and a week later you find yourself at 76mg/dl. and feeling fine. Two days later you are 86mg/dl. after exercise and you are really feeling hypoglycemic symptoms. What I am getting at here is that no one has one number at which they will always feel okay if above and hypoglycemic if below. The number always fluctuates up or down somewhat due to variations in physiological conditions.

One advantage of feeling symptoms at slightly higher numbers, still below 100mg/dl. but above 70 or 75mg/dl., is that it can be treated before it gets low enough to make you feel really bad, before you start feeling even more of the symptoms.

Typical symptoms of hypoglycemia include shaking or trembling, sweating, change of mood (you may get real cranky), headache, a pounding or racing heart, a feeling of weakness or being lightheaded, and a change in vision. You do not have to experience all of these symptoms in order to be hypoglycemic. Also, having more symptoms does not necessarily correlate with how low the blood glucose has gotten. You should immediately stop whatever you are doing and check your blood glucose as soon as you suspect you are hypoglycemic. You may be someone who does not exhibit all of the classic symptoms but may have some that are unique to you.

A very useful and general rule for someone with diabetes, is that whenever you feel peculiar, check your blood glucose. Sometimes a person may suspect they are hypoglycemic because of the way they feel, only to find that when they test their blood glucose to see just how low they are, much to their surprise, they are high. I had a patient in class one time stop me and ask me if I could get her some juice or something because she thought her blood glucose was getting low. I asked her to check her blood glucose while I went to get her some juice. When I returned less than a minute later I saw her standing by her seat looking puzzled. "Never mind," she told me, "My blood sugar is 186. I don't know what's going on, I feel like I'm low."

Some of the symptoms of hypoglycemia may feel similar to symptoms of hyperglycemia. As an example, with hypoglycemia weakness is common, a feeling of running out of gas. With hyperglycemia (high blood glucose), fatigue and lethargy are common. Some people may not be able to easily distinguish between the two.

People who have hypoglycemic unawareness, would be wise to check their blood glucose levels far more frequently than those without the condition and certainly before driving or doing anything requiring concentration where the lack thereof would be dangerous. For those with this condition, checking 6-10 times a day may be necessary. Every case is different, however, so one testing regimen is not right for everyone.

Treatment of Hypoglycemia: When someone is hypoglycemic, it can be very frightening, not just for the patient but for the person treating the patient. With emotions running high, it is very common to over treat. If 4 ounces of soda start bringing the blood glucose levels back up to normal, drinking 8 ounces won't make it happen any faster, and neither will adding a cookie or jelly sandwich. What it *will* do, though, is cause blood glucose levels to be much too high 2-3 hours later.

I live in Florida, and when the air conditioning is not on or not working, in the summer, say in July or August, it can be very, very unpleasant. I remember on one occasion, actually I think it has happened more than once, the air conditioning had not been on for at least several hours and the house was almost 90 degrees. When the air conditioner was turned back on, I noticed a short time later that the thermostat had been pushed all the way to the left as far as it would go. I believe it was set on 60 degrees. I won't say who did it, but it wasn't me. I guess the rationale for doing this was that if the thermostat was turned down to a much cooler temperature, the house would cool off a lot faster. I guess what they didn't understand was that the air that came out of the vents was going to be the same cool temperature whether the thermostat was set at 76 degrees or 60 degrees, and that turning the thermostat down really low was not going to cool the house off any faster.

I guess people who are experiencing hypoglycemia sometimes think that eating a lot of sugar when they are low and feeling poorly, will help them recover faster and feel better sooner. This is very understandable when you consider how poorly most people feel when they are hypoglycemic. I have never heard anyone say they were in pain when hypoglycemic but that it was a very, very unpleasant feeling while it lasted. Similarly the spouse, son, daughter or friend witnessing a hypoglycemic episode can become frightened and encourage taking in more sugar than is needed for the same reasons, that more is better, would work faster and cause the person to feel better more quickly.

The usual treatment for hypoglycemia is to consume 15 grams of carbohydrate when symptoms first begin to appear. If it's possible to check the blood glucose level before taking the 15 grams of carbohydrate, that would be great. If testing the blood glucose is not feasible right then, go ahead with the treatment. If the carbohydrate is in the form of a liquid, it is thought to work faster than if in the solid form. This is probably why orange juice is frequently a treatment of choice. As far as that goes, any fruit juice or even soda is likely to work faster than solids, just hold it to 4 ounces. If you want something besides liquids, there are a lot of other choices. Listed below are just a few.

Name	How many or how much
Life savers	7 or 8, (remember there is a hole in the middle)
Butterscotch or peppermint candy	3-4, (really any hard candy about this size)
Glucose tablets	usually 3-4 depending on the brand
Glucose gel	usually the whole tube, 15 grams
Cake decorating gel	estimate 15 grams
Small piece of fruit	small apple, banana, pear, orange

It is a good idea to stay away from treatments that contain fat as they are not likely to work as fast as treatments made only of sugar. Some would believe that as long as they need to eat something sweet to bring up their blood sugar level, it might as well be something that they really like or yearn for like a Three Musketeers Bar or chocolate covered raisins. Well, I don't blame them, seems harmless enough, but it's really not a good idea. I can think of at least two good reasons why it's not a good idea. The first is that the fat content in the chocolate bar is sky high. This will slow down how fast the sugar enters the blood from the intestinal tract. Secondly, with blood lipid abnormalities and overweight so prevalent in diabetes, few people with the disease can justify eating foods containing this much fat. Most patients I have discussed this with will gladly give up the more desirable sweets for lifesavers or glucose tablets if convinced these treatments will correct their hypoglycemia more quickly.

After treating the hypoglycemia with 15 grams of carbohydrate, it is recommended that you sit quietly and allow the carbohydrate time to get into the blood stream. After 15 minutes, you should check the blood glucose. If the blood glucose level is still less than 100, even when asymptomatic (that means with no symptoms), another 15 grams of carbohydrate should be taken. After taking this second treatment, you should have consumed a total of 30 grams of carbohydrate by now, and glucose levels should not be too low. In some cases they may still be low particularly if too much medication was taken, too much exercise was performed or if a meal was skipped. If any of these are the case, you may want to call your doctor for specific instructions. If an accidental overdose of insulin was taken, the doctor will very likely want to give you detailed instructions.

Accidental overdoses of insulin are not uncommon, particularly when a patient takes two different kinds of insulin. For instance, if the patient is supposed to take 20 units of the long acting insulin glargine before bed and 5 units of quick acting insulin before each meal, gets confused and reverses the directions, taking 20 units of the quick acting insulin before dinner and 5 units of the long acting glargine before bed, this patient is going to become hypoglycemic after dinner. This is also sometimes referred to as insulin shock. In this situation the patient may need to check blood glucose levels and eat some carbohydrate hourly until the blood glucose looks as though it is going to stabilize at a safe level.

Assuming a medication error is not the cause of the hypoglycemia, once the blood glucose level is up above 100 if a meal is not in the immediate future, like within the next hour, it would be wise to have a small snack to sustain the blood glucose level until the next meal.

In the event of an unexpected hypoglycemic episode, which could happen to anyone taking a cheerleader medication or insulin injections, it is a good idea to always keep a treatment for hypoglycemia with you. Lifesavers or hard candy is good for this because they don't melt. I recommend anyone with diabetes always keeping something sweet with him or her because you just never know.

Hypoglycemia Treatment for Someone Unconscious: It is always advisable to treat and get hypoglycemic events under control as quickly as possible. Not only does it feel crummy to be low but ignoring or minimizing early symptoms could lead to a much more serious situation, that being unconsciousness.

Once someone has lost consciousness, levels of glucose in the blood are so low that the brain is not getting the glucose it needs to function properly. Even though most people survive with no serious repercussions after losing consciousness, as far as we know, it is something you want to avoid. After all what if you were in the bathroom taking a shower or driving a car when you passed out? Falling in the shower, that's not a good thing, and neither is losing consciousness while driving. That could easily be fatal.

It is always a good idea to let relatives, friends and people you work with know what to do in the event you ever lose consciousness in front of them or if they come into a room and find you unconscious. This is particularly true if you become hypoglycemic often or have lost consciousness before due to hypoglycemia or take insulin. Not knowing how to deal with an unconscious hypoglycemic patient can be very dangerous and result in death.

If someone were to lose consciousness due to hypoglycemia while in the presence of someone else, the person witnessing the collapse should quickly call 911 or the emergency medical services. They should then return and place the victim in what is known as the recovery position. This position puts the victim on their side with the upper leg bent, preventing the victim from rolling all the way over onto their stomach. The caregiver should stay with the victim, ensuring that they do not roll over onto their back.

The reason for the recovery position and one reason for staying with the victim is that when the victim regains consciousness there is a good chance they will vomit. They don't always vomit but they do enough to make it a concern. In this position if the person vomits, the contents of the stomach will spill onto the floor, and the victim is not likely to choke. If the person is lying on their back and vomits, the stomach content can go down the windpipe and into the lungs, resulting in aspiration pneumonia or choking to death. Under no circumstances should any food, liquid or gel be placed in the victim's mouth when they are unconscious. In most cases, the victim regains consciousness in a matter of a few minutes. This is because in each of our bodies we have a protective mechanism that is activated when the blood glucose level gets dangerously low. When blood glucose levels are too low, the liver releases sugar that has been stored in the liver into the blood.

This is usually enough for the victim to regain consciousness but not enough to maintain a safe blood glucose level. Once conscious, if the victim is coherent enough to take small sips of juice, cola, or any drink containing sugar, they should be encouraged to do so. Asking someone incoherent to suck on a piece of hard candy or a Lifesaver could lead to choking and is not recommended. The victim should be fully capable of consuming whatever treatment is given. As soon as it is safe for the victim to drink and chew, they should consume 15 grams of carbohydrate and then have their blood glucose tested after 15 minutes. The treatment recommendations from here on are the same as for someone who is hypoglycemic who is conscious.

The reason for calling 911 or EMS is because they serve as a good backup. If the victim does not regain consciousness in several minutes, or if complications develop as a result of the low blood glucose, EMS is on the way.

Glucagon

A hormone called glucagon is responsible for the sugar being released from the liver when the level of sugar in the blood is too low. In effect, the glucagon is what tells the liver to go ahead and release the sugar into the blood. In some cases, when a patient reports having lost consciousness the doctor will prescribe glucagon.

It can be picked up at the pharmacy with a prescription. Glucagon comes in a syringe ready to administer. The glucagon is not for the patient to use but for the person with the unconscious patient to use on the patient. Did you get that? It works like this. Let's say you are the spouse of someone that has just lost consciousness due to a severe episode of hypoglycemia. You would still call 911, and you would still put the patient in the recovery position. Once that is done, however, you would get the glucagon kit, follow all the directions for reconstituting the glucagon and then inject it as you would insulin into the patient. The glucagon would stimulate the liver to release more sugar into the blood, which in turn should help the patient regain consciousness.

Keeping glucagon on hand is not considered necessary for everyone, and the majority of diabetes patients probably don't even know what it is. It is usually only recommended for those patients who are at high risk for having severe hypoglycemia and losing consciousness.

Sick Day Guidelines

One thing we can always count on is getting sick. Maybe not today, not tomorrow, but it's going to happen. If you are someone who doesn't get sick very often, that's really good, particularly when you have diabetes. This is because when you have diabetes any illness can play havoc with your blood glucose levels and make control more difficult. What happens is that when you are ill, your liver, which I talked about just recently, will release more sugar into the blood. Your body views being sick as stressful, which it is. It is a physical stress on your body.

With significant potential for blood glucose levels to fluctuate, particularly go high, extra attention is needed in taking care of diabetes during times of illness. With this in mind, there are some specific guidelines that have been established and should be followed when sick.

First of all, when sick you should always continue to take your diabetes medication unless your doctor has told you otherwise. This is so important that it bears repeating, so I will. When sick you should always continue taking your diabetes medication unless your doctor has told you otherwise. Failing to take the appropriate amount of diabetes medication when sick is probably one of the biggest mistakes people make that can get them in serious trouble. It is certainly understandable why this mistake is so common. If I didn't have the knowledge I have and was someone with diabetes I imagine I would do the same thing.

This is what often times happens.

Let's say it is you. We'll make it personal. You wake up one morning feeling very sick. Your stomach hurts and you feel nauseated. The smell of food coming from the kitchen makes you feel even worse. You know you can't eat; even if you could you probably couldn't keep it down. What you're probably thinking is, I know that if I don't take my diabetes medication and I eat, my blood sugar is going to be too high, but since I'm not eating, it's okay not to take it. That may be alright if your liver wasn't releasing extra sugar in your blood due to your illness, but unfortunately it is.

Even without breakfast, without putting any food or drink in your stomach since the night before, without your morning dose of medicine, your blood sugars could be in the two or three hundreds. When sick you take your diabetes medication even if you can't eat. If you are uncomfortable with this for any reason, then call your doctor and ask for specific instructions on what to do.

If you are someone who takes insulin, the doctor may tell you to reduce the dosage by a certain amount; however, any instructions like this should come from the doctor. The response to this that I normally get from patients is, "Yes, but if I take my diabetes medicine and don't eat because I'm too queezy, isn't my blood sugar going to drop too low?" My answer to that is maybe. But remember, your blood sugar levels are probably going to be higher than they normally are when you wake up in the morning if you are sick, maybe 100 or more points. It is possible you can get away with very little food intake while sick without blood sugars going too low compliments of the liver releasing sugar into the blood.

Now another important thing to remember when sick is that it is very difficult, if not impossible, to predict what blood sugar levels will do when sick. We know the blood sugar levels are likely to rise but can't say that for sure. This brings me to the next very important recommendation.

Check blood glucose levels more often than usual while sick.

In some situations, as an example, if you have a major infection, fevers, or are taking steroid medications, it may be necessary to test the blood sugar levels every two to three hours.

Believe it or not, they could change a lot in 2-3 hours. When blood sugar levels rise above 250 mg/dl. for any two consecutive readings, in a two to three hour period of time, calling the doctor for specific instructions on what to do is recommended. How often you test your blood sugar when not sick has no bearing on how often you test when you are sick.

Let's say that you also have diarrhea and are vomiting. Then another concern would be dehydration.

I have seen patients with diabetes get themselves in big trouble because they didn't respond as needed to all of the vomiting they were doing. The same is true for uncontrolled diarrhea. That would be in contrast to controlled diarrhea, which I don't think there is such a thing. Anyway, the point is that their blood sugars got way out of whack, as well as their hydration status after a day of frequent vomiting with nothing to eat, and they ended up in the ICU that evening. About 24 hours later, I interviewed the patient and he was quite surprised how a day of nausea and vomiting could have messed him up so bad.

If vomiting continues and cannot be controlled, meaning you cannot keep anything down, the doctor should be notified. The doctor may be able to stop the vomiting by prescribing a medication.

Earlier I mentioned that you might get by with little food for a while when you have some kind of stomach ailment or, say, food poisoning, from a blood sugar prospective that is. However, if there is vomiting, diarrhea, or both, dehydration becomes a real problem and you need to make sure you replace the fluid you lose with fluid ingested. For this reason primarily, I recommend that you always keep your favorite soda, Gatorade or popsicles in your refrigerator or freezer respectively. I'm talking about a soda with real sugar in it and popsicles sweetened with real sugar. Assuming you cannot eat as you normally would due to nausea, etc., you should try taking small sips of your soda or small bites of your popsicle until they are gone. By doing this, you are helping to maintain a normal hydration level. Once they are gone, start another one. I'm not suggesting you drink three or four 12 ounce Cokes by noon, however. What we are trying to accomplish by drinking something with real sugar in it instead of something sugar free is that we are trying to replace some of the carbohydrates that would have been taken in at breakfast.

The same is true with lunch. A usual lunch for you, if you weren't sick, might contain 45-60 grams of carbohydrates. If you are not up to your usual lunch, you could try a liquid lunch that may be more easily tolerated by your stomach. Theoretically, your liquid lunch could contain the same amount of carbohydrate as your usual lunch. The overall goal here, actually two goals, are to ingest something that you can keep down and prevent dehydration and to replace some of the carbohydrate that you would have consumed if you were eating the way you normally do when not sick. Eating or drinking to accomplish these goals is known as a sick day meal plan. What is chosen to eat or drink is up to the patient and usually depends on what foods the patient can tolerate.

Some examples include any soft drink with real sugar, Gatorade or other electrolyte replacement drink, Jell-O, popsicles, pudding, broth, freeze pops and saltines.

As soon as the illness starts to improve and the patient can return to more normal eating habits they should do so and eliminate the foods and drinks they had been consuming while sick.

From everything I have written in this section regarding illness it may seem as though I am only concerned with ailments that cause you to vomit or have diarrhea, illnesses that involve the stomach or intestinal tract. Any illness, whether it involves the stomach or not, is likely to raise the blood sugar and temporarily affect blood glucose control. An abscess on the big toe can raise blood sugars to the same extent as a stomach virus. I tend to emphasize the illnesses that can cause vomiting and diarrhea because of the tendency to complicate the illness by causing dehydration.

Let's review for a minute. Key points to remember when sick:

1. **Always take diabetes medication.** Blood sugar levels are likely to be higher when there is some kind of infection. If uncomfortable taking the normal dose because you are afraid that your blood glucose level may drop too low, consult your doctor.

2. **Check blood glucose levels more frequently when sick.** Blood sugars are more likely to fluctuate when there is an infection. If above 250mg/dl. on two consecutive readings, contact doctor for instructions.

3. **Follow sick day meal plan, just mentioned.** Goals are to replace fluids lost through vomiting and diarrhea to maintain normal state of hydration and, secondly, to provide the body

with the glucose that would have been provided if regular meals could have been eaten.

Foot and Skin Care

When you have diabetes, you need to take very good care of your feet. When you have diabetes you need to take very good care of your feet. You notice how I wrote that twice? I did it for effect. I sometimes do that when I am writing about something that is really important. People with diabetes are much more likely to have wounds that are slower to heal. For this reason, precautionary measures need to be taken to avoid incurring an injury of any sort to the feet and lower legs. Blisters, spider bites, ant bites, bee stings, ingrown toe nails, cuts and abrasions can all turn into very serious problems if not cared for properly. Keep in mind that germs love your blood, probably more than the blood of other people you know.

What makes your blood so special? It's got a lot of sugar in it. It's a great place for germs to multiply, rapidly. The blood may not circulate down there in the feet as well as it should either. Remember it's not unusual to have impaired circulation when you have type 2 diabetes.

Did you know the leading cause of non-traumatic amputations is diabetes? Of the patients I have seen who have undergone an amputation, I would guess that at least 50 percent of them, and probably more like 75 or 80 percent could have prevented it.

Imagine how you would feel if you lost a limb, say your lower leg, because you kept postponing going to the doctor for treatment, or thought you could take care of the wound without the doctor's help. You didn't want to waste the doctor's time with such a small wound, or you felt silly going to the doctor with a handful of big welts on your foot as a result of ant bites.

By adhering to the following guidelines as well as taking good care of your feet, in general, any serious complications concerning the feet should be avoided.

1. Always wear shoes. Even in the house it's a good idea, particularly when in the kitchen cooking or cleaning up. A patient called me not long ago to tell me she would not be in to exercise for the next couple of weeks because she dropped a can on her toes while in the kitchen, and her foot was hurting her pretty badly. I asked her if she had shoes on; she paused, and sounding somewhat embarrassed replied, "no." The way I look at it is that the best way to ensure your wounds will heal properly is to avoid getting them.

2. Inspect your feet daily. We learn what a normal foot looks like fairly early in life. By taking the time to inspect your feet daily you can identify early on when something doesn't look right, if a blister is forming, if a corn or bunion is starting to show up, etc.

3. After inspecting your feet, if something doesn't look right, contact your doctor. What unfortunately happens is that people wait until the wound gets much worse before finally seeing a doctor. In some of these cases the patient has waited so long before deciding to see a doctor that the likelihood of the patient having a good outcome is slim.

4. Trim your toenails straight across. This reduces the chances of developing in grown toenails. Sometimes toenails can get a little out of control if left untrimmed. If regular nail clippers are not sufficient to get the nails trimmed, see a podiatrist. Avoid going to the shed and pulling out the rose clippers or grabbing a pocketknife. It's been done. It's a good way to cut yourself and end up with an infection.

5. Avoid wearing tight socks that leave an indentation around your calf or ankle. You want to avoid anything that restricts the blood flow to your feet. Circulation to the feet can become impaired with diabetes, and you don't want to do anything to restrict it further. There are specially made socks that don't have seams for people with diabetes.

6. Do not soak your feet. Taking a tub bath is okay as long as you use warm water and not hot water, by the way, when running a bath. The main point here is that you do not want to purposely go soak your feet in a solution of any kind. An exception to this is if your podiatrist (foot doctor) prescribes it with specific instructions. Soaking your feet can dry them out, encouraging the skin to crack.

7. Pedicures are strongly discouraged. Pedicures are discouraged for a lot of reasons. Not only do they involve soaking your feet, but also, do you know how well the little tubs you put your feet in are cleaned between clients? What about the tools used to work on your feet? Are they adequately cleaned? I have heard from many patients that when they have a pedicure, the pedicurist uses a razorblade to shave off calluses, corns, dead skin, etc. Never let anyone that is not a medically trained professional come anywhere near your feet with any kind of cutting instrument.

8. Never put lotion between your toes. Most any good moisturizing lotion can be used on your feet to help keep them moist, but under no circumstances should you let the lotion get between your toes. The reason for this is that when your feet sweat during the day, there may end up being too much moisture between the toes, which increases the chances of developing a fungal infection between the toes and under the toenails.

9. Always check the inside of your shoes before putting your feet in them. This is particularly true if you have neuropathy and diminished feeling in your feet. When there is a partial or total lack of feeling in the feet, you could slip your foot into a shoe that has a small rock or pebble in it and not even notice it. After walking around with a rock or pebble in your shoe all day, you may notice some cuts, abrasions or bruises on your foot.

A Diabetes Holiday

A diabetes holiday now and again shouldn't be a problem. A diabetes vacation, now that could be a different story. Aside from not having diabetes at all, someone with diabetes would like nothing more than to take some time off from having diabetes. I have never really posed this question to a patient of mine, but I believe my statement to be true. The rigors of successfully managing diabetes day after day can take their toll. Taking a day or two off and living it up a bit once in a while might not be too harmful, particularly if you don't throw all caution to the wind and go off the deep end with your eating. Indulging yourself once in a while sounds very reasonable. The key things to remember here are **don't overindulge your indulgences** and **once in a while**, not weekly.

Don't misunderstand me here. I am not encouraging you to stray from good diabetes care; I am simply saying that **once in a while** straying a little bit, say because you are celebrating a special occasion or something, is probably not such a bad thing, particularly if you do it infrequently and get back on track immediately. As much as you might like to take an extended vacation from your diabetes and forget about it for a week or so, I wouldn't recommend it.

There are drawbacks to taking a diabetes holiday besides the temporary increase in blood glucose levels. The first being you might like doing it so much that you start doing it too often. Also, in some cases it might take a day or so after the holiday to get blood glucose levels back to where you want them. Some people find that once they are in the habit of doing something such as eating better or exercising regularly it is much easier just to keep doing it than to make a change every so often like taking a day off. I guess what it all comes down to is what works for you.

In Conclusion

When I sat down to write this book I had no idea how long it would be. I knew what I wanted to accomplish. I knew the major points I wanted to make and that explaining the value of exercise and encouraging patients to give it a try was my first and foremost goal, for I knew that if I could persuade patients to start exercising regularly, their diabetes control would be almost instantly better. I wanted to keep the book simple and not go into too much detail except when necessary. Sometimes big thick books with small print and a lot of graphs and tables can be intimidating. Well maybe not for you but it is for me. I purposely wanted to keep my book relatively short, including only a small number of graphs and charts. I didn't want to throw in any more medical terms than necessary. I wanted the book to be one I might read if I hadn't written it.

So if after reading the book it seems to you as though there is a disproportionate emphasis on exercise relative to nutrition and medication, you are right, there is. That is exactly what I want you to notice. I'm sure there are some good books on the market today that explain how to manage type 2 diabetes; however, I am doubtful that any will encourage exercise to the extent that I have in this book. It has been my experience that when it comes to managing diabetes, the emphasis is always on what you should and should not eat and taking your medications. That's why I needed to write this book.

Now that it is written and I am all but finished, I will leave you with one last thought. I'm sure at one time or another you have been watching television or been at the movies and watched a scene where one character grabs another character by the shoulders during a time of crisis and shakes them, shouting something like this, " Calm down, calm down, get a hold of yourself. You have got to listen to me! Listen to me!" the character yells.

The character who was near hysterics calms down enough to listen to the words of wisdom about to be spoken from the man doing the shaking. (At this point imagine that you are the hysterical person and I am the person with wisdom that shook you. This is what I say to you.). "You have got to start exercising. Don't wait another day. Please, before it's too late."

Glossary

1. Exercise

Planned structured and repetitive bodily movement done to improve or maintain one or more components of physical fitness. 1,2

2. Physical activity

Bodily movement that is produced by the contraction of skeletal muscle and that substantially increases energy expenditure.1,2

3. Physical fitness

a set of attributes that people have or achieve that relates to the ability to perform physical activity.1,2

4. Blood pressure

The pressure exerted by the blood against the vessel walls, especially the arteries.

5. Total cholesterol

The total of the high density and low density cholesterol, plus triglycerides and Lp(a) cholesterol. ADA

6. HDL cholesterol	About one-fourth to one-third of blood cholesterol is carried by high-density lipoprotein (HDL). HDL cholesterol is known as "good" cholesterol, because high levels of HDL seem to protect against heart attack. ADA
7. LDL cholesterol	Low-density lipoprotein (LDL) cholesterol is known as the "bad" cholesterol. When too much LDL (bad) cholesterol circulates in the blood, it can slowly build up in the inner walls of the arteries that feed the heart and brain ultimately leading to a heart attack or stroke. ADA
8. Lp(a) cholesterol	A genetic variation of LDL (bad) cholesterol. A high level of Lp(a) is a significant risk factor for the premature development of fatty deposits in the arteries that ultimately lead to a heart attack or stroke. ADA
9. Triglycerides	Triglycerides are a form of fat made in the body. They can be elevated for a variety of reasons including being over fat or obese, a lack of physical activity, cigarette smoking, excess alcohol consuming too many carbohydrates (greater than 60 percent of total calories). People with high triglycerides often have a high total cholesterol level, including a high LDL (bad) level and a low HDL (good) level. Many people with heart disease and/or diabetes also have high triglyceride levels. ADA

10. Pancreas

The pancreas is about a six inch long organ that has two major roles. It makes enzymes that are necessary for the digestion of food in the small intestine and it is where you will find the "Islets of Langerhans", specialized clusters of cells, including beta cells, responsible for the manufacture and release of insulin.

11. Beta cells

cells are located within the "Islets of Langerhans", responsible for the manufacture and release of insulin into the blood.

12. Insulin Resistance

Insulin Resistance Insulin resistance is a condition that often leads to type 2 diabetes and continues even after diabetes is diagnosed. When insulin has a harder time than usual getting the doors to the muscle, fat and liver cells open allowing the sugar to enter the cells, this is called insulin resistance.

13. Peripheral neuropathy

Peripheral neuropathy is a form of nerve damage that is estimated to affect approximately fifty percent of people with diabetes. Symptoms can include tingling, burning, painful throbbing, weakness and numbness. Peripheral neuropathy is usually first noticed in the feet and lower legs and in some cases followed in the hands.

14. Autonomic neuropathy	Autonomoic neuropathy affects the nervous system (ANS). The ANS controls functions in our bodies that are not under conscious control. This includes regulating body temperature, digestion, heart rate and blood pressure responses to exercise, bladder control, the intestinal tract, dilatation of the retina to light, the genitals, and other organs.
15. Diabetic retinopathy	Diabetes retinopathy is damage to the retina usually caused by chronically elevated blood There are four stages of diabetic retinopathy ranging from mild to proliferative that ultimately can lead to partial or total blindness.
16. Nephropathy	The kidney is made up of little structures known as nephrons that filter waste from the blood. Nephrons have a rich supply of tiny blood vessels that can become damaged when blood sugar levels are high. When the nephrons become damaged they lose their ability to filter waste from the blood adequately and as a result protein can leak into the urine.
17. Isles of Langerhans	Specialized clusters of cells, including the beta cells that make insulin, located in the pancreas.

18. Impotence

Impotence can be defined as the inability to maintain an erection long enough for sexual intercourse, and, or the inability to achieve ejaculation.

19. Capillaries

Capillaries are the smallest blood vessels in the body that carry blood. A dense cluster of capillaries is referred to as a capillary bed.

20. Peripheral nerves

Peripheral nerves are billions of nerve cells that run throughout the entire body that transmit information to the brain as well as other parts of the body. The brain and spinal cord are not part of the peripheral nervous system.

21. Hypoglycemia

Hypoglycemia occurs when blood glucose levels fall below 100mg/dl. and physical symptoms of hypoglycemia are present. Classic symptoms of hypoglycemia include but are not limited toshaking, sweating, irritability, a rapid pounding heart beat and headache.

22. Aerobic exercise

Exercise that utilizes the larger muscles of the body in a continuous, rhythmic manner over a sustained period of time that leads to increased oxygen and heart rate levels.

23. Anaerobic exercise

Anaerobic exercise is exercise that is performed in short, non continuous bouts that is not dependent on increases in oxygen supply.

24. Lean tissue

Lean tissue is muscle.

25. Adipose tissue

Adipose tissue is fat.

26. Body composition

Body composition refers to the amount of fat and muscle in the body and their proportion to one another, often referred to as a percentage of one to the other.

27. Max. heart rate

Max. heart rate is the maximum rate at which the heart can beat when performing a vigorous activity. This can be determined by noting the failure of the heart rate to rise with an increase in workload.

28. RPE scale

RPE scale stands for Ratings of Perceived Exertion scale. This is a scale that is used to subjectively measure how hard it is to perform a given amount of work. This scale can be used alone or in combination with other methods of determining exertion levels

References

1   Diabetes: Heart Disease and Stroke (n.d.). Retrieved 12/13/07 from http://www.diabetes.org/heart disease-stroke.jsp

2   Diabetes Risk Assessment (n.d.). Retrieved 12/13/07 from http://www.Clevelandclinic.org/ health/interactive/diabetes. swf

3   LeRoith, D. The Link Between Insulin Resistance, Metabolic Syndrome, and Cardiovascular Disease, (2006). Oral presentation, University Community Hospital, Tampa, FL

4   Diabetes Control and Complications Trial. (1993). The *New England Journal of Medicine*, 329(14), 1035-1036.

5   American Diabetes Association: Clinical Practice Recommendations 2006. (2006). Standards of Medical Care, Position Statement. *Diabetes Care*, Volume 29, supplement 1, S-11.

6   Tour of the Basics (2007). The University of Utah, Genetic Science Learning Center. Retrieved 12/13/07 from http://www.learn.genetics.utah.edu/

7   Marchand, L., (n.d.). The Pima Indians: Obesity and Diabetes. Retrieved 12/13/07 from http:// www.diabetes.niddk.nih.gov/dm/pubs/pima/index.htm

8   Eaton, B. (2006). Healthy Biological Heritage versus Culturally Related Pathology. American College of Sports Medicine 53rd Annual Meeting, June 1st, 2006, Denver, Colorado.

9   American Diabetes Association: Clinical Practice Recommendations 2006. (2006). Standards of Medical Care, Position Statement, *Diabetes Care*. Volume 29, supplement 1, S- 5.

10 American Diabetes Association: Clinical Practice Recommendations 2006. (2006). Standards of Medical Care, Position Statement. *Diabetes Care*, Volume 29, supplement 1, S-10.

11 Day, A. *Good Dog Carl*. (1997). Simon and Schuster Children's Publishing.

12 Unpublished data. (2003). Diabetes Care Institute.

13 Hagberg, J.M. (2005). Exercise your way to lower blood pressure. *American College of Sports Medicine*, brochure, Retrieved 12/13/07 from http:// www.***acsm***.org.

14 Whelton, S.P., Chin, A., Xin, X., & He, J. (2002). Effect of Aerobic exercise on blood pressure: A meta analysis of Randomized, Controlled Trials, *Annals of Internal Medicine*, 136(7), 493-503.

15 Blumenthal, J.A., Sherwood, A., Gullette, E.C.D., Babyak, B., Waugh, R., Georgiades, A., et al. (2000). Exercise and weight loss reduce blood pressure in men and women with mild hypertension. *Archives of Internal Medicine*, 160: 1947-1958.

16 LaForge, R. (n.d.) Managing Cholesterol with Exercise. Retrieved 12/13/2008 from http:// ***www.acefitness.org/ fitfacts/fitacts***.

17 Mueller, J. (2005). Heart-Healthy Benefits of Exercise.. Retrieved 12/13/07 from http:// ***www.sparkpeople.com/ resource/health***

18 Kravitz, L., & Heyward, V. (1994). The Exercise and Cholesterol Controversy. Retrieved 12/20/07 from http://*www.Unm.edu/~lKravitz/Article*

19 Milvy, P. (1977). The Marathon: Physiological, Medical, Epidemiological, and Psychological Studies. *Annals of the New York Academy of Sciences*, 301(1), 346-360, New York, NY.

20 Holme, I. (1991). An analysis of randomized trials evaluating the effect of cholesterol reduction on total mortality and coronary heart disease incidence [published erratum, *Circulation*, 84(6), 2610-1].

21 Heaner, M. (n.d.). Good cholesterol, bad cholesterol, can exercise make a difference? Retrieved 12/13/2007 from http://*msn.health.com/centers/cholesterol.*

22 Nash, T. (2004). Cardiovascular risk beyond LDL-C levels; Other lipids are performers in cholesterol story. *Postgraduate Medicine*,116(3).

23 Safeer, R.S. & Ugalat, P.S. (2002). Cholesterol Treatment Guidelines Update, *American Family Physician*. 65(5), 871-880.

24 Durstine, J.L., Pate, R.R., Sparling, P.B., Wilson, G.E.,Senn, M.D., & Bartoli, W.P. (1987). Lipid, lipoprotein and iron status of elite women distance runners. *Int. J Sports Med,* 8(suppl 2), 119-123.

25 Gibbons, L.W., Blair, S.N., Cooper, K.H., & Smith, M. (1983). Association between coronary heart disease risk factors and physical fitness in healthy adult women. *Circulation*, 67: 977-983.

26 Couillard, C., Despres J.P., Lamarche, B., Bergeron, J., Gagnon, J., Leon, A.S., (2001). Effects of endurance exercise training on plasma HDL cholesterol levels depend on levels

of triglycerides: Evidence From Men of the Health, Risk Factors, Exercise Training and Genetics (Heritage) Family Study. *Arteriosclerosis, Thrombosis, and Vascular Biology,* 21:1226-1232.

27 Kodama, S., Tanaka, S., Kazumi, S., Miao, S., Sone, Y., Onitake, F., & Sone, H. (2007). Effect of Aerobic Exercise Training on Serum Levels of High-Density lipoprotein Cholesterol. A Meta analysis. *Archives of Internal Medicine,* 167: 999-1008.

28 Despres, J., Tremblay, A., Nadeau, A., & Bouchard, C. Physical training and changes in regional adipose distribution. (1988). *Acta Med Scand Suppl.* 723: 205-212.

29 Barret-Connor, E., Slone, S., Greendale, G., Kritz-Silverstein, D., Espeland, M., Johnson, S.R., et al. (1997).The Postmenopausal Estrogen/Progestin Interventions Study: primary outcome in adherent women. *Maturitas,* 27(3), 261-274.

30 Tall, A. (1990). Plasma high density lipoproteins: metabolism and relationship to atherogenesis. *J Clin Invest.* 86(2), 379-384.

31 Racette, S. B., Schoeller, D.A., Kushner, R.F., & Neil, K.M. (1995). Exercise enhances dietary compliance during moderate energy restriction in obese women. *Am J Clin Nutr.* 62: 345-9.

32 Ross, R., Janssen, I., Dawson, J., Kungl, A., Kuk, J., Wong, S., et al. (2004). Exercise- Induced Reduction in Obesity and Insulin Resistance in Women: a Randomized Controlled Trial. *Obesity Research,* 12: 789-798.

33 Duncan, G., Perri, M., Theriaque, D., Hutson, A., Eckel, R., & Stacpoole, W. (2003). Exercise training, without weight loss, increases insulin sensitivity and post heparin plasma lipase activity in previously sedentary adults. *Diabetes Care,* 26: 557-562.

34 Pan, X., Li, G., Hu, Y., Wang, J., An, Z., Hu, Z., et al.(1997). Effects of diet and exercise in preventing NIDDM in people with impaired glucose tolerance. The Da Qing IGT and Diabetes Study. *Diabetes Care*, 20(4), 537-544.

35 Lindstrom, J., Louheranta, A., Mannelin, M., Rastas, M., Salminen, V., Eriksson, J., Uusitupa, M., and Tuomilehto, J., for the Finnish Diabetes Prevention Study Group. (2003). The Finnish Diabetes Prevention Study (DPS): Lifestyle Intervention and 3-Year Results on Diet and Physical Activity. *Diabetes Care*, 26(12), 3230-3236.

36 Ross, R., Dagnone, D., Jones, P., Smith, H., Paddags, A., Hudson, R., Janssen, I. (2003). Does exercise without weight loss improve insulin sensitivity? *Diabetes Care*, 26: 944-945.

37 Pate, R., Pratt, M., Blair, S., Haskell, W., Macera, C., Bouchard, C., et al. (1995). Physical activity and public health: a recommendation from the Centers for Disease Control and Prevention. *JAMA*, 73(5), 402-407.

38 Abstract. American College of Sports Medicine. JAMA 273: 422-407, 1995

39 Blair, S., Kohl, H 3rd., & Barlow, C. (1995). Changes in physical fitness and all- cause mortality: a prospective study of healthy and unhealthy men. *JAMA*. 273: 1093-1098.[Abstract].

40 Ekelund, Ulf., Franks, P., Sharp, S., Brage, S., & Wareham, N. (2007). Increase in physical activity energy expenditure is associated with reduced metabolic risk independent of change in fatness and fitness. *Diabetes Care*, 30: 2101-2106.

41 Weiss, E.P., Racette, S.B., & Villareal, D.T. (2006). Improvements in glucose tolerance and insulin action induced by increasing energy expenditure or decreasing energy intake: a randomized controlled trial. *Am J Clin Nutr*. 5: 1033-42.

42 Weiss, E.P., Racette, S.B., Villareal, D.T., Fontana, L., Steger-May, K., Schechtman, K., Klein, S., Holloszy, J., and the Washington University School of Medicine CALERIE Group l. (2006). *Am J Clin Nutr*. 84(5), 1033-42.

43 Goodpaster, B. American Diabetes Association research profile (November 2004).

44 Snowling, N., & Hopkins, W. (2006). Effects of Different Modes of Exercise Training on Glucose Control and Risk Factors for Complications in Type 2 Diabetic Patients: A meta-analysis. *Diabetes Care*. 29: 2518-2527.

45 The Diabetes Prevention Program (DPP) Research Group. The Diabetes Prevention Program (DPP). (2002). Description of lifestyle intervention. *Diabetes Care*, 25: 2165-2171.

46 Bassuk, S. & Manson, J. (2005). Epidemiological evidence for the role of physical activity in reducing risk of type 2 diabetes and cardiovascular disease. *J of Appl Physiol*. 99(3), 1193-204.

47 American Diabetes Association: Clinical Practice Recommendations 2006. (2006). Standards of Medical Care, Position Statement. *Diabetes Care* (29), supp.1, S-14.

48 Fowler-Brown, A., Pignone, M., Tice, J.A., Pletcher, M., Sutton, S.F., Lohr, K.N., et al. (2004). Exercise Tolerance Testing to screen for coronary heart disease: a systematic review for the technical support for the U.S. Preventive Services Task Force. *Ann Internal Med*. (140): W9-W24.

49 U S Preventive Services Task Force. (2004). Screening for coronary heart disease: recommendation statement. *Ann Intern Med*. 140: 569-572.

50 U S Department of Health and Human Services. (1996). Physical Activity and Health: A Report of the Surgeon General. Atlanta GA, U S Department of Health and Human Services,

Centers for Disease Control and Prevention, National Center for Chronic Disease Prevention and Health Promotion.

51 Pate R., Pratt M., Blair S., Haskell, W., Macera, C., Bouchard, C., et al. (1995). Physical activity and public health. A recommendation from the Centers for Disease Control and Prevention and the American College of Sports Medicine. 273(5), 402-407.

52 Albright, A., Franz, M., Hornsby, G., Kriska, A., Marrero, D., & Ulrich, I. (2000). The American College of Sports Medicine Position Stand. Exercise and Type 2 Diabetes. *Med Sci Sports Exerc.* 7: 1345-60.

53 Dunstan, D., Daly, R., Owen, N., Jolley, D., de Courten, M., Shaw, J., et al. (2002). High-intensity resistance training improves glycemic control in older patients with type 2 diabetes. *Diabetes Care*, 25: 1729-1736.

54 Castaneda, C., Layne, J., Munoz-Orians, L., Gordon, P., Walsmith, J., Foldvari, M., et al. (2002). A randomized controlled trial of resistance exercise training to improve glycemic control in older patients with type 2 diabetes. *Diabetes Care*, 25: 2335- 2341.

55 Ibanez, J., Izquierdo, M., Arguelles, I., Forga, L., Larrión, J., García-Unciti, M., et al. (2005). Twice-weekly progressive resistance training decreases abdominal fat and improves insulin sensitivity in older men with type 2 diabetes. *Diabetes Care*, 28: 662-667.

56 Camps, K. Being Active. (n.d.). The Art and Science of Diabetes Self- Management Education: A Desk Reference For HealthCare Professionals; Section 3; Facilitating Successful Self-Management; Chapter 30; Knowledge Publication. The American Diabetes Association of Diabetes Educators, Publisher.

57 Whaley, M.H., Brubaker, P.H., & Otto, R.M., eds. (2006). American College of Sports Medicines *Guidelines for Exercise Testing and Prescription*, 7th ed. Baltimore, Md: Lippincott Williams & Wilkins.

58 Kaminsky, L.A., Bonzheim, K.A., Garber, C.E., Glass, S.C. et al, eds. (2005). American College of Sports Medicine. *Resource Manual for Exercise Testing and Prescription*, 5th ed. Baltimore, Md: Lippincott Williams & Wilkins.

59 Karvonen, M., Kentala, K., & Mustala, O. (1957). The effects of training on heart rate: a longitudinal study. *Annales Medicinae Experomentalis et Biologial Fennial*, 35: 307-315.

60 Kolata, G. (2001, April 24). Maximum heart rate theory is challenged. *The New York Times*, Health Page.

61 Kolata, G. (2003). *Ultimate Fitness: The Quest for Truth About Exercise and Health*, Douglas & McIntire.

62 Borg, G. (1998). *Borg's Perceived Exertion and Pain Scales.* (Figure 7.3, page 49) Human Kinetics.

63 Wing, R.R., Blair, E.H., Bononi, P., Marcus, M.D. Watanabe, R., Bergman, R.N. et al. (1994). Caloric restriction per se is a significant factor in improvements in glycemic control and insulin sensitivity during weight loss in obese NIDDM patients. *Diabetes Care*, 17: 30-36.

64 Kelley, D.E., Wing, R., Buonocore, C., Sturis, J., Polonsky, K., & Fitzsimmons, M. (1993). Fitzsimmons M. Relative effects of calorie restriction and weight loss in patients with non-insulin dependent diabetes mellitus. *J Clin Endocrinol Metab.* 77: 1287-1293.

65 Franz, M.J. (2003). Diabetes Management Therapies: a Core Curriculum for Diabetes Education; Chapter 1, Medical Nutrition Therapy for Diabetes: Fifth Edition, Chicago, Illinois.

66 Summary of the second report of the national Cholesterol Education Program (NCEP) Expert Panel on Detection, Evaluation, and Treatment of High Blood Cholesterol in Adults. (1993). *JAMA*, 269: 3015-3023.

67 Haffner, S.M. (1998). Management of dyslipidemia in adults with diabetes (technical Review). *Diabetes Care*, 21:160-178.

68 Garg A. (1998).Treatment of diabetic dyslipidemia. *Am J Cardiol.* 81:47B-51B.

69 Quest Diagnostics Inc.(2007).

70 Smith. S.C. Jr., Blair, S.N., Criqui, M.H., Fletcher, G.F., Fuster, V.,Gersh, B.J. et al. (1995). Preventing heart attack and death in patients with coronary artery disease. [American Heart Association consensus statement]. *Circulation*, 92: 2-4.

71 Franz, M.J. Protein controversies in diabetes.(2000). *Diabetes Spectrum*, 13: 132-141.

72 Nuttall, F.Q., Mooradian, A.D., Giannon, M.C., et al. (1984). Effect of protein ingestion on the glucose and insulin response to a standardized oral glucose load. *Diabetes Care*, 7: 465-470.

73 Gannon, M,C., Nuttall, F.Q. (2001). Effect of protein ingestion on the glucose appearance rate in people with type 2 diabetes. *J Clin Endocrinol* Metab. 86: 1040-1047.

74 American Diabetes Association. Evidence- based nutrition principles and recommendations for the treatment and prevention of diabetes and related complications (position statement). (2003). *Diabetes Care*, 26(suppl 1), S51-S61.

75 Hunt, I. & Spinney, R. (2006). Organic Chemistry On-Line Learning. Retrieved 2/06/08 from http:// www.chem.ucalgary.ca/courses/351/Carey5th?Ch25/ch25- 1-2.htm.

76 Nuttall, F.Q., Gannon, M.C., Franz, M.J.,Bantle, J.P., eds. (1999). Carbohydrates and Diabetes. *American Diabetes Association Guide to Medical Nutrition Therapy for Diabetes*, Alexandria, Va: American Diabetes Association. 107-125.

77 Franz, M.J., Bantle, J.P., Beebe, C.A., Brunzell, J.D., Chiasson, J. L., Abhimanyu, G., et al. (2002). Evidence-based nutrition principles and recommendations for the treatment and prevention of diabetes and related complications (technical review). *Diabetes Care*, 25: 148-198.

78 US Department of Agriculture and US Department of Health and Human Services. (2000). Nutrition and Your Health: Dietary Guidelines For Americans 2000. 5th ed. Hyattsville, Md: USDA Human Nutrition Information Service; Home and Garden Bulletin No. 232.

79 Tuck, M., Corry, D., & Trujillo, A. (1990). Salt-sensitive blood pressure and exaggerated vascular reactivity in the hypertension of diabetes mellitus. *Am J Med*. 88: 210-216.

80 The sixth report of the Joint National Committee on Prevention, Detection, Evaluation and Treatment of High Blood pressure. (1997). *Arch Intern Med*. 2143-2446.

81 Sacks, F.M., Svetkey L.P., Vollmer, W.M., Appel, L.J., Bray, G.A., Harsha, D., et al. (2001). Effects on blood pressure of reduced dietary sodium and the Dietary Approaches to Stop Hypertension (DASH) diet. *N Engl J of Med*. 344 (1), 3-10.

82 Markovic, T.P., Jenkins, A.B., Campbell, L.V., Furler, S.M, Kraegen, E.W., Chisholm, D.J. (1998).The determinants of glycemic responses to diet Restrictionand weight loss in obesity and NIDDM. *Diabetes Care*, 21: 687-694.

83 UK Prospective Diabetes Study (UKPDS) group. (1990). UK Prospective Diabetes Study 7: response of fasting plasma glucose to diet therapy In newly presenting type 2 diabetic patients. *Metabolism*, 39: 905-912.

84 Yeh G, Eisenberg D, Kaptchuk T, Phillips, R.S. et al. (2003). Systematic Review of Herbs and Dietary Supplements for Glycemic Control in Diabetes. *Diabetes Care*, 26: 1277-1294.

85 Mukamal, K.J., Conigrave, K.M., Mittleman, M.A., Camargo, C.A. Jr., Stampfer, M.J., Willet, W.C. et al. (2003). Roles of drinking pattern and type of alcohol consumed in coronary heart disease in men. *N Eng J Med*. 348: 109-118.

86 Wei, M., Gibbon, L.W., Mitchell, T.L., Kampert, J.B., & Blair, S.N. (2000). Alcohol intake and incidence of type 2 diabetes in men. *Diabetes Care*, 23: 18- 22.

87 Sacco, R.L., Elkind, M., Boden-Albala, B., Lin, I.F., Kargman, D.E., Hauser, W.A. et al. (1999). The protective effect of moderate alcohol consumption on ischemic stroke. *JAMA*, 281: 53-60.

88 Bell, R.A., Mayer-Davis, E.J., Martin, M.A., D'Agostino, R.B., & Haffner, S.M. (2000). Association between alcohol consumption and insulin sensitivity and cardiovascular disease risk factors: the Insulin Resistance and Atherosclerosis Study. *Diabetes Care*, 23: 1630-1636.

89 Davies, M.J., Baer, D.J., Judd, J.T., Brown, E.D., Campbell, W.S., & Taylor, P.R., (2002). Effects of moderate alcohol intake on fasting insulin and glucose Concentrations and insulin sensitivity in post menopausal women. *JAMA*, 287: 2559-2562.

90 Valmadrid, C.T., Klein, R., Moss, S.E., Klein, B.E., & Cruickshanks, K.J. (1999). Alcohol intake and the risk of coronary heart disease mortality in persons with older-onset diabetes mellitus. *JAMA*, 282: 239-246.

91 Solomon, C.G., Hu, F.B., Stampfer M.J., Colditz, G.A., Speizer, F.E., Rimm, E.B., et al. (2000). Moderate alcohol consumption

and risk of coronary heart disease among women with type 2 diabetes. *Circulation*, 102: 494-499.

92 Ajani, U.A., Gaziano, M., Lotufo, P.A., Liu, S., Hennekens, C., Buring, J., et al.. Alcohol consumption and risk of coronary heart disease by diabetes status. *Circulation*, 102: 500-505.

93 National Cholesterol Education Program Expert Panel on Detection, Evaluation, and treatment of High Blood Cholesterol in Adults: Executive Summary of the Third Report of the National Cholesterol Education Program (NCEP). Expert Panel on Detection, Evaluation and Treatment of High Blood Cholesterol in Adults (Adult Treatment Panel III) (2001). *JAMA*, 285: 2486-2497

94 What is avandia? (1997-2007). Retrieved 12/13/2007 from http:// www.avandia.com.

95 What is Actos? (1999). Retrieved 12/15/2007 from http:// www.actos.com.

96 Franz, M. (2003). *Diabetes Management Therapies: a Core Curriculum for diabetes education*; chapter 3, Pharmacologic Therapies for Glucose Management: Fifth. edition, Chicago, Illinois.

97 Bailey, C. (1993). Metformin: an update. *Gen Pharmacol.* 24: 1299-1309.

98 Wu, M., Johnston, P., Sheu, W., Hollenbeck, C.B., Jeng, C.Y., Goldfine, I.D. et al. (1990). Effects of metformin on carbohydrate and lipoprotein metabolism in NIDDM patients. *Diabetes Care*, (13), 1-8.

99 Authers not listed. (2002). Diabetes Information: Pills. Retrieved 1/24/2008 from http:// www.fda.gov/diabetes/pills.html.

100 Kalberg, J.B., Walter, Y.H., Nedelman, J.R., & McLeod, J.F. (2001). Mealtime glucose regulation. *Diabetes Care*, (24), 73-7.

101 Keilson, L., Mather, S., Walter, Y.H., Subramanian, S., & McLeod, J.F. (2000). Synergistic effects of nateglinide and meal administration on insulin secretion in patients with type 2 diabetes mellitus . *J Clin Endocrinol Metab*. 85: 1081-1086.

102 Ratner, R.E., Dickey, R., Fineman, M., Maggs, D.G., Shen, L., Stroebel, S. et al. (2004). "Amylin replacement with pramlinitide as an adjunct to insulin therapy improves long-term glycaemic and weight control in type 1 diabetes mellitus: a 1- year, randomized controlled trial". *Diabetes Med*, 21 (11), 1204-1212.

103 Kruger, D., Gatcomb, P., Owen, S., Van Rossum, D., Menard, D.P., Fournier, A., Et al. (1999). Clinical implications of amylin and amylin deficiency. *Diabetes Educ*. 25(3), 389-397. PubMed Abstract

104 Young, A.A., Vine, W., Gedulin, B.R., Pittner, R., Janes, S., Gaeta, L.S.L., et al. (1996). Preclinical pharmacology of pramlinitide in the rat: Comparisons with human and rat amylin. *Drug Development Research*, 37: 231-248.

105 Learn about Symlin. (2007). Retrieved 1/22/08 from http://www.symlin.com.

106 Mcintyre, N., Turner, D.S., & Holdsworth, C.D. (1964). New interpretation of oral glucose tolerance. *Lancet*, 41(2), 20-21.

107 Elrick, H., Stimmler, L., Hlad, C.J., & Arai, Y. (1964). Plasma insulin responses to oral and intravenous glucose administration. *J Clin Endocrinol Metab*, 24: 1076-1082.

108 Creutzfeldt, W., & Ebert R. (1985). New developments in the incretin concept. *Diabetologia*, 28: 565-573.

109 Supplement to The Diabetes Educator. Vol 32: supplement 2:68S March /April 2006.

110 Drucker, D.J. (2003). Enhancing incretin action for the treatment of type 2 diabetes. *Diabetes Care*, 26: 2929-2940.

111 Kreymann, B., Williams, G., Ghatei, M.A., & Bloom, S.R. (1987). Glucagon- Like peptide-1 (7-36): a physiological incretin in man. *Lancet*, 2: 1300-1304.

112 Komatsu, R., Matsuyama, T., Namba, M., Watanabe, N., Itoh, H., Kono, N., et al. (1989). Glucagonostatic and insulinotropic action of glucagon-like peptide 1–(7-36)-amide. *Diabetes*, 38: 902-905.

113 Gutzwiller, J.P., Goke, B., Drewe, J., Hildebrand, P., Ketterer, S., Handschin, D. et al. (1999). Glucagon-like peptide-1: a potent regulator of food intake in humans. *Gut*, (44), 81-86.

114 Authors not listed. (2008). For healthcare professionals: Explore the possibilities. Retrieved 1/2/2008 from http:// www.januvia.com.

115 Retrieved 12/01/2007 from http:// www.phytomedical.com/ Diabetes/Timeline.asp.

116 Sattley, M. (1996). Diabetes Timeline. Retrieved 10/15/2007 from http:// www.diabeteshealth.com/read/1996/11/01/714. html.

117 Authors not listed. (2007). How LANTUS® Works: Long-Acting Insulin MOA Retrieved 2/07/2008 from http://www. lantus.com/hcp/works.aspx.

118 Homko, C., Deluzio, A., Jimenez, Jerzy, W. Kolaczynski, and Boden, G. (2003). Comparison of Insulin Aspart and Lispro: Pharmacokinetic and metabolic effects.

119 *Diabetes Care*, 26: 2027-2031. 119 Roenstock, J., Schwartz, S.L., Clark, C.M., Park, G.D., Donley, D.W., and Edwards, M.B. et al. (2001).Basal insulin therapy in type 2 diabetes. 28 week comparison of insulin glargine (HOE 901) and NPH insulin. *Diabetes Care*. 24: 631-636.